Praise for *How to* *Stay Stopped for G*

'To say I was pessimistic about my chances is putting it mildly – I thought I'd be the last man on earth to be able to stop smoking. I had tried in vain to quit a few times until I finally stopped in the summer of 1997 with the guidance of Gillian Riley.'
MARK KNOPFLER, MUSICIAN

'In my experience, Gillian Riley's method is the only one (of many I have encountered) that really gets to the heart of the addiction and roots it out. I feel so much better for not smoking, and have gained no weight as a result. I'd strongly recommend her technique to anyone who is serious about getting free of this addiction.'
JULIET STEVENSON, ACTRESS

'I have found it a very helpful resource for my work in running stop smoking groups in general practice. The philosophy is not only straightforward but also it works.'
JULIE BROMILOW, PRACTICE NURSE, LONDON

'I am so relieved to be free from my nicotine prison that it's like being reborn. Having your book near me was like having a personal friend to lean on who understood my addiction.'
ANNE WILSON, HOUSEWIFE, BELFAST

'What impressed me at the time was the elegant simplicity of your solution. It seemed to capture the right amount of information necessary to make the final push for quitting. I believe many people totally underestimate the psychological side of nicotine addiction. I congratulate you on a cohesive integration of all the relevant ideas.'
JOHN GAFFNEY, LECTURER IN PSYCHOLOGY, SLIGO, IRELAND

'I stopped smoking three years ago after reading your book. Your approach hit the right spot in my imagination, removing the anxiety out of the process – after nearly 30 years of being a roll-up smoker.'
MARTIN GODLIMAN, VIOLIN MAKER, MIDDLESEX

'My involvement with this approach has been both personal and professional. Six years ago, after being a smoker for 25 years and having tried every other conceivable method of stopping smoking, I discovered this technique. Not only was it a successful and painless method but it explained in a rational way the psychology of addiction. I believe every doctor who is responsible for advising smokers would benefit enormously from reading this book and applying its principles. This technique offers a huge advancement in the treatment of nicotine addiction.'
DR SIMON MCMINN, GENERAL PRACTITIONER, CHELTENHAM

'I believe there is a special way in which your method allows the fact of not smoking to integrate its way into one's life. The reason for this lies in one simple notion – that of choice. I know that every previous attempt to stop smoking on my part was characterised by lack of choice and sooner or later "freedom" would assert itself and I would be back smoking again.'
JULIAN GILMORE, UNEMPLOYED, KENT

'When I realised that the amount of money my husband and I were spending on cigarettes was more than our mortgage repayments, I decided to buy your book. Reading it thoroughly and regularly helped me to stop, and I managed, a week after giving up, to take and pass my driving test without worrying about cigarettes. I have been a successful ex-smoker for over three years now. Although I tried a couple of times, I have never before had this success with giving up. My husband is still on 60 a day and I am happy to have him smoke in front of me. A totally excellent book – worth its weight in gold.'
LOUISE CRITCHELL, HOUSEWIFE AND MOTHER, DORSET

'Two pages in and I was hooked. It all began to make sense and what a help it has been and will be in our work. The book is proving invaluable both to us and to our groups. It is top of our reading list. Many thanks again for producing such a helpful guide.'
SHIRLEY MARQUIS, HEALTH PROMOTION ADVISER, BLACKPOOL

'Straightforward and simple, it succeeds without drugs, hypnotism or acupuncture. It worked for me after all other "treatments" had failed within a few days. I find it still hard to believe that after 40 years of smoking latterly 40 cigarettes a day, now, years later, I feel not so much of a twinge let alone a puff! It really works!'

DR ANTHONY FLOOD, MC, CONSULTANT PSYCHIATRIST, CUMBRIA

'I was as heavy a smoker as you can imagine. I remember trying to give up once and then scrabbling through a bin the next morning desperately searching for my cigarettes. Your book made me realise that if I made a real choice I could give up. I do not think I could have stopped without it.'

RICHARD PARKER, TEACHER, NORTH LONDON

'I had stopped smoking for about six months and was nearly "cracking up" when I discovered your book. You saved my sanity! I couldn't lend it to anyone as I needed to know it was there all the time for reference. It is now four years and five months since I stopped and I'm very proud. No one should attempt to stop smoking without reading your book and learning about the psychology of addiction. I want to encourage people to have a go; it's such a relief to leave it behind! No more chest infections, no more cough medicine and neither of my children have needed antibiotics for four years.'

CHRISTINE JOHNSTON, MOTHER AND STAFF NURSE, MIDLOTHIAN

'Her techniques are refreshingly free from gimmickry and seem to be well founded psychologically. If her impressive figures can be replicated elsewhere, the Full Stop Programme could represent a breakthrough in preventative medicine.'

MEDICAL MONITOR

'The Outline offers a clear and simple choice which makes a lot of sense to my clients, whether from the shop floor or the chief executive's office. This approach offers neither a magic wand nor a quick fix: it can take time for individuals to alter strongly held attitudes and beliefs about their own smoking. But once they understand they have the freedom to choose, the sense of deprivation disappears and the experience of quitting becomes both positive and liberating.'

GILLIAN GRAVESON, SMOKING CESSATION CONSULTANT, GLASGOW

'You do not have to avoid your usual work patterns, pleasures or other smokers ... life does not change in any way except for not smoking. I started out sceptical, ended up very impressed and now I recommend the course to patients. I think the technique is good because neither drugs nor much willpower is required.'
GENERAL PRACTITIONER

'For 25 years I smoked 20+ cigarettes a day and for the latter 15 of those years I wanted to give up. There were many occasions that I attempted to stop, with success that ranged from a few hours to as long as 12 months. During those times, however, I was continually desperate for a cigarette and spent an enormous effort fighting the addiction. It wasn't that I didn't want to give up enough or that I lacked the willpower. The problem was wasting energy on a powerful addiction without any strategies that could help. Then I read this book, followed the suggested method, and had my last cigarette – four years ago. Although I found it difficult initially, unlike previous attempts, it became easier with time. Whereas before I had always denied the craving which of course just kept returning, this method helped me to face and deal with my addiction, which allowed me to take control of my life. Now quite honestly I find it hard to believe that I was a smoker for all those years.'
SANDY PRESSDEE, STUDENT, BOURNEMOUTH

HOW TO STOP SMOKING AND STAY STOPPED FOR GOOD

Fully revised and updated

GILLIAN RILEY

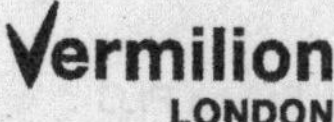

9 10 8

First published in the United Kingdom in 1992 by Vermilion
This edition published in 2007 by Vermilion, an imprint of
Ebury Publishing

Ebury Publishing is a division of the Random House Group

The Random House Group Limited Reg. No. 954009

Addresses for companies within the Random House Group can be found at www.randomhouse.co.uk

A CIP catalogue record for this book is available from the British Library

ISBN 9780091917036

The Random House Group Limited supports The Forest Stewardship Council® (FSC®), the leading international forest-certification organisation. Our books carrying the FSC label are printed on FSC®-certified paper. FSC is the only forest-certification scheme supported by the leading environmental organisations, including Greenpeace. Our paper procurement policy can be found at www.randomhouse.co.uk/environment

Printed and bound in Great Britain by Clays Ltd, St Ives PLC

Contents

Foreword

Stopping smoking is like a journey from safe shores into uncharted waters, leaving behind established routines for a profoundly healthier lifestyle – but never far away is the risk of failure and a return to old habits. Having the courage to attempt this is important but not enough, which is why 90 per cent fail and return to smoking. What is also needed is a map of how to get there, listing pitfalls and hazards along the way.

We have been running smoking cessation clinics twice weekly for many years and used various behavioural techniques including hypnosis, relaxation training and stimulus control. None of these methods answered the important questions patients put to us.

Gillian Riley at last provided us with the answers; not complicated, theoretical ones, but simple solutions that all our smokers could relate to. Her innovative technique, developed through years of counselling smokers, provides a completely new look at smoking and is very different from established methods. Established techniques relying on aversion or avoidance failed many of our clients. This technique works because it explains the truth about smoking and enables smokers to live with their feeling of wanting to smoke and thereby control their addiction.

I strongly recommend this book to smokers and all health workers, who will find it as helpful as I did in many areas of their work.

Dr A. N. Sherwood
King's Lynn, Norfolk

Smoking Cessation Team of the Year Award, Doctor *magazine*

Action on Smoking and Health/British Heart Foundation Award

Preface

Anyone who has ever wanted to stop smoking has dreamed of a magic cure – an easy, effortless solution that takes the whole problem away. Smokers often want to find a way to stop and never doubt their decision, never feel tempted to smoke again and therefore never fear failure.

Most therapies and techniques encourage this dream. Those people who threaten, needle, shock and hypnotise smokers into stopping focus on a process that reinforces the decision to quit, promising permanent success if this first step is taken.

But it is one thing to stop smoking and quite another thing to stay stopped. In one article, a hypnotist claims a 90 per cent success rate. Another, in his book, claims that 80 per cent succeed with his methods. But neither gives any reference to how long these ex-smokers remained 'cured'. Five minutes? Five weeks? Without that information, these claims are virtually meaningless.

According to research at the University of London (published in the medical journal *Addiction* in 2005) more than 85 per cent of smokers who have given up return to smoking within a year.

Perhaps you could say that if these people go back to smoking later on, it's their own fault. But could it be that there are crucial flaws in the techniques employed; flaws that will inevitably lead the great majority of ex-smokers back to their old ways?

How to Stop Smoking and Stay Stopped for Good regards stopping smoking not as an event, but as part of a process. The process begins even before stopping and continues for some time after the last cigarette has been extinguished.

This is because stopping smoking is really about changing the way you think about smoking. It's a matter of becoming aware of the kind of thinking that supports the addiction, and resolving the conflicts it creates. And that doesn't happen in an instant, like magic.

For you, this is both good news and bad news. The bad news is that it's not just a matter of deciding to stop and toughing it out for a few days. Most smokers have already done that at some time and still gone back to smoking after weeks or months of abstinence.

The good news is that if you recognise and understand the mental aspects of the addiction, you have a far greater chance of long-term success than if you try to pretend that it isn't there.

Every smoker is different, but they all have much in common: a powerful, insidious and often underestimated drug addiction. If you cannot grasp how this addiction works, no amount of motivation or willpower will enable you to succeed in the long term.

Stopping smoking is the first giant step, but it's not just a matter of stopping. It's learning the skill of staying stopped that's the real challenge. And that's what this book is all about.

Part One
Understanding Addiction

CHAPTER 1

How to Use This Book

Our remedies oft in ourselves do lie
Which we ascribe to heaven.

WILLIAM SHAKESPEARE, ALL'S WELL THAT ENDS WELL

The technique that this book describes is radically different from any other you will have come across. Although the message may at times seem obvious, in practice it requires a change in your mental approach that needs to be worked at. It will challenge the way you have been thinking about smoking and will require you to question and absorb completely new ideas. This takes time, and the most valuable thing you can do is to make stopping smoking the number one priority in your life while you are going through this major change.

The way to learn this technique is to read this book thoroughly, frequently and, most important of all, privately. As far as possible, tell no one that you are thinking about stopping smoking, don't discuss what you are doing in the process of stopping, and try to keep quiet for as long as you can about having stopped, when you do. This may seem unusual, but there are some very good reasons for doing it this way.

It's not that your smoking doesn't affect other people, because it does. And it's not that other people aren't entitled to their opinion about your smoking, because they are. The reason it's best to keep it to yourself is because the first step for you in taking control of your smoking is to recognise that your smoking is a problem *you* have created, and it's *your* problem to solve.

If you keep this technique private, you will learn to rely completely on yourself, and therefore you will be able to stay stopped, no matter who is or isn't with you. It can make the difference between success and failure if you can remember that whether you smoke or not is entirely up to you. It will also help you to stop smoking – and stay stopped – because *you* want to, and not to please others.

If friends or family know you are reading this book, tell them you don't want to discuss it. The whole process of stopping smoking will be, and needs to be, on your mind a lot to begin with, so it can be very tempting to keep talking about it. But if you do, you will invite their comments, and encouragement and advice from other people can so easily end up feeling like pressure or nagging.

I think that you will understand more clearly the value of keeping this private as you read on, but it's important to put this into practice from the beginning.

If you and your partner both want to stop, my advice is not to stop smoking at the same time. You can get competitive, resentful of each other's failure or success, and your own motivation can get tied up with wanting the other to succeed. If you do stop smoking at the same time as a partner or friend, at least don't discuss it at all during the first few weeks.

You might believe it's impossible for you to stop smoking unless your partner or friend stops as well. But you will find, as many others have, that one of the best things about this technique is that you will have no difficulty spending time with other smokers after you have stopped.

You might, however, want to create or join a support group, or have one person, a counsellor for example, to talk things through with. This won't counteract the benefit of keeping the process private if you make sure you discuss stopping smoking only with that group or person, and *only* at specific times. This is entirely different from talking about stopping at home, during work or on social occasions with anyone who will listen.

If you do use a group or support person, make sure they don't have a vested interest in you stopping smoking. In other words, if someone in your life has been pushing you to stop smoking, they are not the person to ask for support.

And it's going to be helpful for the person or people supporting you to be familiar with this technique. Otherwise, they will inevitably advise you in ways that are contrary to this approach.

How much time you spend reading and at what point you stop smoking is entirely up to you. You might read this book through once and feel inspired to stop immediately. Or it may be that it won't start to make any real sense until you have read it through a number of times.

If someone in your life has been pushing you to stop smoking, they are not the person to ask for support.

This has very little to do with how intelligent you are and a great deal to do with how addicted you are. Because the central ideas require a complete revision of your habitual way of thinking, it might take a while for you to really understand them.

If you think that a particular chapter has just clicked something vital into place in your mind, whether it's on your first reading or your twentieth, by all means go ahead and stop smoking there and then. If you decide to stop during your first read, make sure that you are able to finish the whole book as soon as possible, because there will almost certainly be some crucial information for you in each chapter.

If, however, you get to the end and still don't feel ready to stop, then I suggest that you read and reread, and then set a target date for stopping. Write it down, with a specific time, so that you don't conveniently 'forget' it; and keep working with the technique to overcome your resistance to making the necessary changes in the way you think.

This book will act as your support system, so it's very important that you continue to read it once you have stopped, and keep coming back to review what you have read for weeks and even months after.

Hang on to your own copy of this book, underline things and write comments for yourself: the more you get involved with it, the more real it will become to you and the more likely you are to succeed long term.

Part One will introduce you to the ideas behind the technique and why it works. Part Two focuses more on how to put it all into practice. The index will help you locate specific information you may want to review. The section at the end called 'Your Plan For Stopping' provides a step-by-step guide that summarises the whole process. At the end of each chapter are contributions from people who have attended my course, describing in their own words how this technique worked for them.

Throughout the book I have referred exclusively to the activity of smoking cigarettes. This is out of brevity and because the vast majority of those addicted to nicotine take their drug in this form. Exactly the same technique applies, however, to anyone wanting to take control of nicotine addiction in any form, including cigars, pipes, snuff, chewing tobacco, and nicotine replacement products, such as gum.

Is there a right time to stop smoking? Only you will know when that moment will be. It's best not to choose a time of great stress. If you use this technique correctly, the process of stopping will require your attention to begin with. You will need to spend some time studying this book and thinking about what you are doing. So, if you have something unusual and particularly demanding coming up soon, such as exams, it's better to wait until after they are over before you go ahead with stopping smoking. If you are in an unusually traumatic situation, for any reason, it will be better to wait a while.

The sooner you stop, the better.

If you have recently stopped taking some other drug you have been dependent on, whether prescribed or not, it will be advisable to wait a while before stopping smoking, *especially* if you increased your level of smoking in the process. You will have transferred at least some of your dependency over to cigarettes, and you may be taking on too much at once to try stopping smoking as well. If you want to stop taking another drug but have not yet done so, then it's fine to stop smoking first: just deal with each problem one at a time.

Apart from these circumstances, the sooner you stop, the better it will be for you. You are the only one who can decide whether you have a really justifiable reason to wait or if you are just making excuses.

It might be a good idea, right now, to write on the inside front cover the date you bought or started to read this book. Then, if you pick it up again much later on, and you still haven't got around to stopping, you may get stunned into action!

IN OTHER WORDS: JEAN

What I want to say to people reading this book is don't worry about it, just read it – it makes sense. Even if you don't manage to stop, you will always remember key things which, when you do give up, will be invaluable.

I had no expectations when I started the course. I had smoked for nearly 30 years. I had tried acupuncture and hypnotherapy, both of which only helped me to cut down for a brief time. I smoked 30 a day, which I enjoyed, and really never wanted to give up. I hoped for a miracle and a magic wand, which I also knew did not exist.

The most important thing to learn was to stop smoking for myself. I spend my life doing things for others (as most women do) and didn't think to do something for me. This has changed my life.

you will always be "busy"
Are you just making excuses
so you don't have to quit?

CHAPTER 2

The Nature of Addiction

A cigarette is the perfect type of a perfect pleasure. It is exquisite, and it leaves one unsatisfied. What more can one want?
OSCAR WILDE

When I was a smoker, I didn't think of myself as addicted. I just thought I was smoking, like most other people I knew. It was only when I stopped smoking and was seriously trying to stay stopped that I began to realise that I had, in fact, been in the grip of an addiction.

Often smokers deny they are addicted even though they smoke daily for years. You hear them say: 'I'm not addicted – I enjoy smoking,' as if the two were mutually exclusive. These are the smokers who claim they can stop easily any time they want to. But, you may notice, they don't stay stopped.

Other smokers are all too eager to admit to being addicted because they use that to justify their smoking. Being addicted is their way of explaining – to both themselves and others – why they continue to smoke, with the implication, of course, that there is nothing they can do about it.

Then there are smokers who take such a severe moral stance towards any drug addiction that they are very reluctant to think of themselves in that way. These people have a stereotyped image of the 'drug addict' as a deviant and dangerous character. Each drug addiction has its own unique qualities, but just because a drug is legal doesn't mean that it isn't just as addictive as one that is illegal. Millions of people have become dependent on relatively socially acceptable drugs such as nicotine, sugar and caffeine.

So what is an addiction? Is it in your mind or in your body? And what can you do about it? Understanding addiction, and especially this one, is your first step.

Nicotine in Your Body

Here is an important question to consider. If you have found stopping smoking to be intolerable, or if you find you can stop but you keep going back, is this because your body has developed a need for nicotine, a physical dependency that must be satisfied at any cost? Let's start by looking at what happens in your body and in your mind when you smoke.

First and foremost, smoking a cigarette is a way of administering the drug nicotine. Some gets absorbed slowly through the inside of your mouth but most of it is inhaled into your lungs where it is very rapidly taken into your blood stream. It is then carried in the blood all round your body, and especially to your brain.

Many people think that the reason they smoke is to maintain the amount of nicotine in their blood. This, they think, is what drives them to light cigarette after cigarette. However, if you carefully examine your own experience of smoking, I think you will see there is actually something else far more important to you.

Look at it this way. What if, unknown to you, somebody, somehow, put nicotine into your blood stream. Would you really have any way of knowing it was there? And, even more important, would you then lose your desire to smoke?

I think you would still want to smoke, for the same reason that you sometimes still want to light up another cigarette even when you've just finished one. For the same reason that people still crave cigarettes while they are chewing nicotine gum. A number of scientific experiments demonstrate this point.

These smokers still wanted to smoke – and did smoke – regardless of whether or not they had adequate amounts of nicotine in their blood stream.

In one, smokers who had abstained from smoking overnight were given an intravenous injection. On one occasion it contained saline and on another it contained sufficient nicotine to reach concentrations in the blood stream comparable to those achieved by smoking. They were not told which was which. 'Subjects were unable to discriminate between conditions. At the end of the infusion there was no difference in self-reported desire to smoke, nor in latency to lighting up a cigarette when this was permitted. Complete nicotine replacement was therefore not accompanied by complete suppression of smoking behaviour.'[1]

These smokers still wanted to smoke – and did smoke – regardless of whether or not they had adequate amounts of nicotine in their blood stream.

The Buzz

Does this mean that nicotine is irrelevant? Certainly not! The point I am making is that when you smoke a cigarette, it's not so much the amount of nicotine in your blood that you want or think you need: you can hardly tell it's there.

What you really want are the sensations you get, for just a few seconds, when a dose of nicotine is *entering* your body. You know the feeling. For a moment your heart races and you feel a dizzy kind of intoxication. Extra adrenalin runs through your body. It's a feeling of excitement, a very brief 'lift' or 'high'. It's a nicotine buzz.

In the experiment I just mentioned, the nicotine was delivered gradually, over one hour. If it had been administered quickly the subjects would have been aware of it and it would have felt to them like smoking, delivering a buzz and thus satisfying their desire to smoke.[2]

If you have ever tried using nicotine replacement products, such as gum, patches or lozenges, you will know what I'm talking about. It delivers the nicotine too slowly to be truly satisfying. Some people can get a very mild buzz from it, and can even get hooked on it, just as some get hooked on other slow-delivery methods, like non-inhaling pipe and cigar smokers. Nicotine in your blood, even if delivered very gradually, will make your heart beat a little bit faster, among other things, but the effect it has is much more subtle. *For the vast majority of cigarette smokers, the buzz is the most important thing, and you only get that from a sudden, rapidly absorbed dose of nicotine.*

Unfortunately this increased heart rate isn't real energy – otherwise athletes would smoke during marathons. It's a false stimulation, and like all artificial highs it's immediately followed by a depressed state. To make matters worse, cigarette smoke includes many poisons too, so although the heart is beating faster there is less energy-producing oxygen in the blood. This is why most smokers find they have *more* energy when they've stopped.

Getting it Right

As you know, the buzz is stronger when you haven't smoked for a while. It's at its best when a dose of nicotine rapidly enters a brain and body that contain relatively low levels of nicotine. Like the first cigarette of the day, for example.

But the balance has to be right, because for most smokers, if you smoke too infrequently the sensations are too strong and can even make you nauseous. So you need to keep smoking a certain amount in order to maintain some tolerance.

On the other hand, if you smoke too frequently you don't get enough buzz. This is the bad news: the buzz is subject to 'rapid acute tolerance'. This means that after the first puff of the first cigarette you've had in a while, you get a much weaker sensation. Quite probably, most of the cigarettes you smoke in a day don't manage to deliver a good buzz, but you keep trying anyway. I know I did.

This is the reason why smokers can still have a desire to smoke even though they've got plenty of nicotine in their body. For some smokers there are times when smoking a cigarette doesn't satisfy the desire, so that they still feel a craving while actually smoking. That's because they are still wanting the buzz but just not getting it. For some this can develop into chain-smoking, which is a continuous and largely unsuccessful attempt to satisfy their desire to smoke.

It's a never-ending tease, delivering the prize just often enough to keep you interested. You try to get that buzz feeling as often as you can, waiting in between cigarettes for as long as possible for the nicotine level to drop a bit, so that it feels strong enough when the nicotine goes in. This is why cigarettes are particularly enjoyable after physical exercise and after a meal: the nicotine level has been brought down, giving you a better buzz when you smoke.

Need or Desire?

The crucial point to understand about the buzz is that it is desired and pursued, consciously or unconsciously, *regardless of how much nicotine you have in your body*. The experience of a client of mine illustrates this vital point.

Malcolm, in his mid-forties, came to one of my courses and told me that six months earlier, quite out of the blue, he had suffered a major heart attack and had been taken to hospital for emergency surgery.

He stayed in the hospital for a week, and although he had been smoking 40 cigarettes a day for 30 years, he hardly even thought of cigarettes while he was there. He told me he didn't feel any withdrawal symptoms and didn't have any particular interest in smoking at all. Of course, he was under some kind of sedation for the first day or two, which would have masked any symptoms he might otherwise have had, but not for the rest of that week.

Then he told me what happened on the day he was discharged. As he walked away from the hospital, he passed a pub and thought how nice it would be to have a beer and a cigarette. So he did, and then he resumed smoking his two packets of cigarettes a day.

The point is that when he went into that pub, it wasn't because his body suddenly wanted or needed nicotine at that precise instant. His body didn't want or need it the day before in the hospital and it didn't then. The reason he smoked was because of the *thought*: 'Wouldn't it be nice to have a cigarette?' which he then acted on. It was a thought he hadn't had for a few days because of the circumstances he was in.

There is an important question here. If Malcolm had not smoked at that time, what would he then have experienced? The answer is that he would have begun the real process of stopping smoking – a process which takes place in the mind – long after the nicotine had left his body.

Malcolm went through the physical stage of withdrawal and didn't even notice it, but he never did go through the psychological withdrawal, and this is why he didn't stay stopped.

The Taste

You may think the reason Malcolm smoked is simply because he enjoyed the taste of tobacco, but this is an effect rather than a cause. Any addict will make positive associations with whatever is directly connected to their addiction. Heroin addicts actually get some satisfaction from injecting themselves with plain water when they can't get heroin. Psychologists call this secondary conditioning.

As a smoker, you develop a special fondness for the taste of tobacco because it has become associated with your nicotine fix. If you only tasted tobacco and never got any buzz at all you would only feel frustrated. I would suggest that the cigarettes you most enjoy – probably only a few in a day – are those that deliver the strongest buzz.

You don't make a positive association with herbal cigarettes because they don't deliver the nicotine buzz. The whole experience of pleasure – the taste and smell, the sensation of the smoke in your throat, the feel and appearance of cigarettes, including your brand logo – is bound up with the one essential component: the buzz.

Physically, nicotine enters the body producing a brief, excited, dizzy sensation, as well as making your heart beat faster for a few seconds. Then, *mentally*, you think: 'That was nice!' or: 'That was helpful!'

The Crutch

'That was helpful!' expresses the common belief that nicotine makes a valuable, even essential, contribution to your life. This belief takes various forms, and you may hold one or more of them yourself:

- You believe that, without nicotine, you will not be as mentally alert, as able to concentrate, or make decisions.
- You think you will not function as well physically, have as much energy, be able to relax completely, get going in the morning, get to sleep at night or digest your food properly.
- You fear you won't be able to control your moods, stay calm or keep anger or depression at bay.
- You are concerned you won't be able to enjoy yourself socially.

These beliefs always look very convincing: they have to be in order to fool you. You would not think, for example, that smoking enables you to leap tall buildings in a single bound. That's too absurd.

The beliefs that smokers develop have to be believable, and even contain fragments of truth. What happens is you take those fragments and go on to ascribe qualities and capabilities to the nicotine far beyond what it actually achieves chemically. After years of living with these misconceptions, eventually cigarettes are thought of as an indispensable crutch.

Discovering what is and isn't true about this so-called crutch is part of what's involved in stopping smoking. In another chapter, 'Why Smoking Seems to Help', we will disentangle the truth from the illusion behind each of these beliefs.

Another word for addiction is dependency: you believe you are dependent on nicotine in order to function as well as you do mentally, physically and emotionally. But no human body actually needs nicotine: your *belief* that you need it – your dependency – is something you can begin to question and re-evaluate as part of the process of stopping.

The Object of Desire

Many smokers, of course, believe themselves to be physically dependent because of the presence of physical withdrawal symptoms whenever they stop smoking. They think they are in for a distressing experience caused by an inevitable, chemical reaction to the absence of nicotine in their system.

The familiar nightmare stories include: tension, restlessness, anxiety, loss of concentration, loss of sleep, hunger, mood changes such as depression, and, last but not least, a dreadful craving for a cigarette. It is, however, a critical mistake to put these distressing effects all down to physical chemistry.

One way to understand the primary cause is to realise that many of these symptoms can be experienced equally strongly in other situations, not connected with chemical withdrawal of any kind. They are, in fact, products of particular *states of mind.*

When it comes to stopping smoking, the attitude you take can either create high levels of tension, anger and anxiety, for example, or it can dispel such negativity, making the process of stopping smoking far more positive and relaxed.

In the same way, your desire to smoke, created by the memory of the nicotine buzz, can either be an intolerable nightmare or an entirely acceptable part of the process, depending on the attitude you take.

Physical Withdrawal

This doesn't mean, however, that everything about stopping smoking is entirely in the mind. Smoking does involve your body, and when you stop there certainly are things that will happen on a purely physical level.

There is a physical withdrawal, which is the result of an inevitable process of change that your body will go through. Along with nicotine, there are in cigarette smoke at least 4,000 different chemicals, many of which are poisonous, that get absorbed into your body. So when you stop, your body goes through a process of recovery: a detoxification.

If you have done a great deal of smoking, it may feel for a couple of days after stopping like you are coming down with a very bad cold. That's about as nasty as it gets. Physical withdrawal is very temporary and not at all dramatic or intolerable. It's actually a cleaning-out process and therefore the beginning of an improved state of health.

After you stop, the nicotine leaves your body. It is eliminated in the same way as any other toxin in the blood stream and, according to medical researchers who have measured nicotine levels in blood samples, it leaves the body *in less than 24 hours.*[3]

The nicotine has an effect on your body, but it's your mind that desires the effect.

Physical damage and residues from many years of smoking will, of course, take longer to rectify, but that is nothing to do with the effects of a drug. If your lungs take a while to clean themselves out, that's just a consequence of having stopped. It's not part of what's involved in being able to stop.

As far as the physical elimination of nicotine is concerned, you don't need to do anything about it. Your body will take care of itself, by itself. Your mind, however, will not!

Addiction in Your Mind

Even after you have stopped smoking and all traces of nicotine have left your body, your memory of smoking still persists. And it is how you handle that memory that primarily affects your experience of stopping smoking – and, most importantly, whether or not you stay stopped.

In fact, what you have done is to form a psychological attachment to the physical sensations you get from smoking. The nicotine has an effect on your body, but it's your mind that desires the effect. It's your mind that believes you need nicotine. It's your mind that registers satisfaction when you get your buzz, or can object in the most dramatic ways if the desire is not satisfied. *And it's your mind that decides whether you'll go on smoking or face the challenge of stopping.*

Physical withdrawal doesn't determine whether you will be successful at stopping smoking. It's your mind that determines whether or not you will go through that experience, and – most crucially – whether or not you go back to smoking, long after those physical changes are over.

When you stop, after some temporary physical changes, your body will be much healthier and happier, since you are no longer putting so much poison into it. But your mind may not be happy because, unlike your body, it does not make the change to not smoking automatically. It remains the mind of a smoker, but it's the mind of a smoker who isn't smoking. And that inevitably sets up a conflict.

All this is the process of the psychological side of withdrawal, and unless it's dealt with correctly you may very well be smoking again weeks or months after the physical withdrawal is over.

If you are still not convinced, it may help to look at other addictions that have nothing to do with the ingestion of a drug. People can become addicted to a whole variety of things, such as gambling, computer games or exercise. These people can experience very similar symptoms when they stop, such as intense compulsions or cravings, feelings of deprivation, anger, irritability, anxiety, depression and panic.

You Can Work it Out

I am not saying that it's all in your mind, therefore you are imagining all your problems and they don't really exist. The problems are real, and so is the addiction.

What I am saying is that in order for you to successfully stop smoking and stay stopped, to really take control of this addiction, you will need to change the way you are thinking about this. And you can't do that by just waiting for it to change: you need to work at it. *It requires your active attention and participation.* This book will show you what to do and why and how to do it. But nobody can change your thinking for you.

An addiction is held in place by an elaborate system of deceptions. If you have been deceiving yourself in this way for a long time, it will probably all look very real to you.

What stopping smoking – and staying stopped – is all about is discovering the truth. Once you have done that, it's not so easy to get conned again. If you are willing to put effort into reading, thinking and questioning, you have every chance of real success this time.

IN OTHER WORDS: DAVID

I had struggled for years with starting and stopping smoking, kidding myself that because I knew I could stop any time I was really in control.

I stopped after my mother died of cancer with a firm intention to stay off. I went back to it a year later and smoked for five years before I stopped again. This time I relapsed after a few months. Then I stopped again, and got back when I allowed myself to smoke a roll-up on the principle that they were different in some way! I was back on 20 a day within a few weeks.

Gillian's course (five and a half years ago) showed me that you can't play with an addiction – it always wins! Now I see it as something with its own power and I know now how to experience an addictive desire, and how to stand outside it without denying it, or feeling denied.

CHAPTER 3

The Desire to Smoke

Tobacco, divine, rare, superexcellent tobacco . . . a sovereign remedy to all diseases. But, as it is commonly abused by most men, which take it as tinkers do ale, 'tis a plague, a mischief, a violent purger of goods, lands, health; hellish, devilish, and damned tobacco, the ruin and overthrow of body and soul.

ROBERT BURTON, *ANATOMY OF MELANCHOLY*

Whenever a thought crosses your mind that leads to the lighting of a cigarette, you have experienced your desire to smoke. Sometimes it feels like an urge, a craving or a compulsion. Sometimes you just think to yourself that you fancy a cigarette, or that smoking would help you in some way. So you light one. As a smoker, you are continuously feeding and satisfying that desire by smoking cigarette after cigarette after cigarette.

A Part of Your Life

The desire to smoke may be associated with virtually any situation or circumstance in your life. This is a feature of all addictions: the conditioned response that the scientist Ivan Pavlov first demonstrated with his dogs. Pavlov rang a bell every time he fed the dogs, and after a while the dogs would salivate whenever they heard the bell, thinking food was on the way. Just like Pavlov's dogs, some smokers actually salivate for a cigarette on hearing the telephone ring. You train yourself, over and over, to expect a cigarette (a nicotine buzz), especially on certain cues.

I'm sure you would have no difficulty in identifying all kinds of things you associate with smoking. This is why smoking is thought of as a habit, because it's so integrated into your life. Just think of all the situations: taking a break, finishing a meal, making a decision, concentrating on a demanding task or just completing one, answering the phone, sitting in a traffic jam, drinking coffee, having a beer, seeing another smoker light a cigarette and smelling the smoke. You will also have conditioned yourself to expect to smoke whenever you feel particular emotions: especially anger and frustration, but also sadness, boredom, anxiety, embarrassment, and even triumph, joy and excitement.

The list is endless. Just about anything that happens, or doesn't happen, in a smoker's life can result in the idea of smoking a cigarette.

Fortunately, it is not essential to identify all these cues, especially since it could be quite an insignificant thought or simply a shift in your thinking, like: 'What shall I do now?' (Answer: 'I'll have a cigarette!') The main point here is that the desire to smoke, the expectation of smoking, is triggered repeatedly. Something happens and you think, automatically, that smoking a cigarette would be helpful and/or enjoyable. So you light a cigarette.

If you've been smoking regularly for a number of years, this thought will be so familiar to you that it can often go unnoticed, such as when you suddenly realise you have a half-smoked cigarette in your hand, with absolutely no recollection of having lit it.

But even though you may not be aware of it, there is *always* something that initiates the lighting of a cigarette. There has to be some impulse that tells your hand to pick up a cigarette and light it. This is your desire to smoke: you just aren't conscious of it at times.

And if you have ever stopped smoking for any length of time, the reason you went back to smoking was because you had that same old desire to light a cigarette, and you did so. Often people say they went back to smoking because of certain circumstances, such as an argument, an accident or a party. But what actually happened was this: the situation triggered a conditioned response – your desire to smoke – which you then satisfied. This may seem obvious, but it's important to see the whole sequence of events: first the cue, then the desire, *then* the action of smoking.

You satisfy the desire, and you reinforce it at the same time.

If you smoke 40 cigarettes a day, then at least 40 times a day you are experiencing – and satisfying – your desire to smoke. Sometimes you enjoy them and sometimes you don't. Sometimes they seem helpful and sometimes they are little more than a nuisance. *Always,* you are smoking not because events somehow magically make you reach out and light up a cigarette, but because they act as a trigger to your addictive desire.

Why do you have this desire to smoke? The answer is simply and entirely because of all the smoking you have done in the past. Smoking is 'learned behaviour'. And you have reinforced your desire to smoke with every cigarette you ever smoked. You satisfy the desire, and you reinforce it at the same time.

If you had only ever smoked ten cigarettes, then your desire to smoke would only have been reinforced ten times. Unfortunately, people who have only smoked ten cigarettes usually aren't motivated to stop smoking. So they go on reinforcing the desire until they have smoked as many as a quarter of a million cigarettes before they really get serious about trying to stop.

Some smokers set up boundaries for themselves, or go along with boundaries set up by others, and don't smoke in certain circumstances. For instance, some people never, ever smoke in certain rooms, such as the bedroom. Others never smoke during breakfast or in their cars, and many never smoke during work situations, such as while teaching, in an office or interviewing people. In these situations, the desire to smoke doesn't usually get triggered because the association either has never been made in the first place or has already been broken. But you are certainly smoking as habitually and addictively at other times.

As we discussed in the last chapter, a desire to smoke is a thought that comes to your mind, regardless of how much nicotine there happens to be in your body at the time. Your body doesn't need more nicotine just because you're on a coffee break. Your body's nicotine level doesn't fall dangerously low the moment a friend comes to visit and lights up in your kitchen. What happens is that you are reminded of smoking when break-time comes along, or the smoking friend shows up, and you anticipate another opportunity to get your nicotine buzz.

Non-smokers and Ex-smokers

What you have done is this: you have trained yourself to

expect a cigarette, especially on certain cues, and you have reinforced that training thousands of times over.

There are people, of course, who never did that. They never smoked, never reinforced the behaviour and so the idea of smoking doesn't occur to them. They are non-smokers, and they often have a hard time understanding why anyone smokes at all. If they get a piece of bad news, they just get upset. They don't get upset and then reach for a cigarette, like you do. Smoking simply doesn't occur to them, not because they were born fundamentally superior in some crucial way, or because their lives are especially easy, but because they never chose to become smokers and establish that particular conditioning in the first place.

The big question here is: is it possible for a smoker to become a non-smoker? Is there a way to stop smoking and never think of smoking again? Can you undo the years of conditioning so that, for example, when the phone rings, you just answer it?

For the great majority of smokers, this looks like the ideal – and perhaps only – solution, but the truth is that once this conditioning has been deeply ingrained, there is no way to magically erase it. It has been too frequently reinforced, too thoroughly integrated into your life and mind. Brace yourself for the bad news: some desire to smoke is likely to recur. However much you may want to forget all about smoking after you have stopped, it's impossible for you to become someone who has never smoked. As a smoker, you cannot become a non-smoker. You can, however, become an ex-smoker. This distinction is crucial.

The good news is that once you have stopped smoking, the conditioned response begins to fade because you are no longer reinforcing it. Provided you handle it correctly, the sooner you stop smoking and the longer you stay stopped, the more it fades. More about this later.

Remembering the Buzz

Once you have become a smoker, you will have a memory of being a smoker. If you can remember things you did only once, 10 or 20 years ago, it's really very likely that you will remember something you did many times, every day, for most of your adult life.

But being reminded of smoking is more than an ordinary recollection, because the nicotine buzz has been etched deep into your memory. It's a memory of the effects of a drug, so it's persistent and feels like desire. If you stop smoking, it will fade gradually, but the old conditioning rarely disappears entirely. This means that even after you've stopped, you will at times still experience some desire to smoke. This will be an automatic reaction, especially on those most significant cues: after a special, celebratory meal, when feeling strong emotions, when in the company of other smokers, to name a few of the most common examples.

This is probably the last thing you want to hear, but, as with any problem, it works much better to tackle the facts rather than pretend they don't exist just because you don't like them.

Most smokers definitely do not like the idea that they may continue to feel the desire to smoke after they have stopped. This is why most stopping-smoking methods are aimed at helping you to avoid this unpleasant reality. You may have tried such a method and found that it helped you to stop – but not to stay stopped.

In the short term, it's relatively easy to focus on the disgusting and dangerous aspects of smoking, so that you are able to fend off the desire to have a cigarette. But it's only a matter of time before that argument wears thin. Your memory of the addiction comes back – you want that buzz – and you are smoking again.

You can learn how to handle this desire without smoking.

A great many smokers, after many failed attempts to stop, have finally come to realise this truth; that the desire is quite persistent, especially for the first few months after stopping. Unfortunately, what they then conclude is that they will not be able to stay stopped for very long. So many smokers fail at stopping smoking over and over again because they are hoping to rid themselves of the addictive desire. *If success for you means never feeling tempted ever again, then failure is inevitable!*

There is, however, a way out. And here is the key. Just because you feel a desire to smoke, *it doesn't mean that you have to smoke.* You can learn how to handle this desire without smoking. You may think, at first, that this is quite impossible, but it is an exceptionally effective approach, and if you are prepared to read on, every step of how to do this will become clear.

I have taught and counselled hundreds of smokers over the past two decades, with excellent long-term results: over 75 per cent of people who completed my course were still not smoking one year later. *To be successful in the long term you will stay stopped not because you have lost the desire to smoke, but because you have learned how to manage it, without smoking.* That's how I have managed to stay stopped, and you can do it too. It takes some time and effort to begin with, but it's possible.

There are two main obstacles to learning how to manage your desire to smoke and so successfully stop smoking. The first is a sense of deprivation, and the second is resisting the desire.

Feeling Deprived

If you've ever stopped smoking in the past and experienced a sense of deprivation, you may also have experienced an aggravated and probably intolerable desire to smoke. Believing you are deprived makes things seem a hundred times worse: you panic, get very intense cravings, and feel depressed, hostile and martyred.

But you can experience a desire to smoke without having a sense of deprivation. You may never have thought that possible, but Chapters 4 and 5 will show you how.

Resisting the Desire

The truth is that, as a smoker, you are faced with two different options. One is to continue smoking. The other is to learn how to deal with your desire to smoke, which enables you to stop and stay stopped.

For many smokers, both these options seem lousy: a lifetime of smoking looks grim, but having an unsatisfied desire to smoke doesn't look much fun either. In fact, once you learn how to manage the desire properly it very quickly becomes easy to live with. But if you don't know how to do this, the best you can hope for is that it will somehow go away if you wait long enough.

If you have ever made any attempt to stop smoking before, you probably know what I'm talking about. It's very likely that you often felt a strong desire to smoke, but tried to ignore it, and at times when that was impossible, you fought it.

This is unfortunate because, in fact, much of the difficulty in stopping smoking comes not from feeling the desire to smoke, *but from not wanting that feeling to be there.* It is because you are setting yourself up in conflict with your desire to smoke that you experience the greatest difficulty. Many symptoms of tension and anxiety – which are thought of as withdrawal symptoms – are a product of this conflict. Nervous energy, nausea, head, jaw, neck, shoulder and stomach aches, clenched teeth and white knuckles are all expressions of a fight going on inside you. It is you fighting your desire, not wanting to feel it. You may not deliberately fight it; this resistance is often automatic.

You may also fear the desire, because while you are in conflict with it, you always feel like you are on the verge of giving in to it. You may feel overwhelmed by it, or fear that you will be overwhelmed by it eventually. The fear makes you fight it even more, so you end up feeling like a battlefield. After a while, when the fighting wears you out, you return to smoking, regretting another failure.

There is, however, a solution to all this. It is highly effective and it's something that can become part of your everyday life. And it has to do with accepting the desire, accepting that it is there, and relaxing with it instead of fighting against it. The desire to smoke is as inevitable as a brick wall. When you stop banging your head against it, wishing it wasn't there, it won't hurt you so much!

There's another problem that comes from resisting the desire to smoke. If you think you should get rid of the desire, you may be able to create the illusion that you have done just that. This is a trap that can make it easy to stop, but is guaranteed to take you back to smoking later on.

At the Back of Your Mind

Most of the time, people who stop smoking see their desire to smoke as their enemy. Mostly they try to ignore it and hope it goes away soon. Some people can shut out the urge completely, so that they don't feel it at all, even in the early stages of stopping. This is called repression.

Repression is a coping mechanism that can be helpful at times. As one very practical example, if you run from danger and sprain an ankle, the pain can often be repressed and only becomes apparent when you reach safety.

Repressing emotions can also be a way of coping with difficult situations. You may repress your anger when an outburst could create trouble. You may repress sadness in order to put on a brave face over some tragedy.

For many smokers, repression of the desire to smoke is the sole mechanism they use to stop smoking. And they are often encouraged to do so, by a broad variety of techniques and books on the subject. Sometimes the advice is directed towards getting smoking off your mind: keep yourself busy, change your routines and avoid situations that might make you want to smoke. If you think about smoking, distract yourself quickly so that you don't feel too tempted.

Some people like to boast about being able to stop without experiencing any desire to smoke at all, or maybe only a little. This just means they are repressing the desire very effectively. Some people repress things easily, some people don't. It doesn't necessarily mean that you are less addicted.

If you stopped smoking in the past and thought it was easy, then you probably did it by repressing. In Chapter 2 we looked at the story of Malcolm, who completely repressed his desire to smoke for a whole week while in hospital. He is not uncommon: many smokers are able to repress for days or weeks at a time, especially when they are ill or in unfamiliar surroundings. But even if you can keep it up for days or weeks, it is rarely possible to repress for ever.

Many smokers are quite unable to repress at all. And many smokers become less able to repress their desire to smoke as the years go by. So, for example, a smoker who can repress effectively after five years of smoking, and so stop smoking for periods of time, will most likely not be able to after 20 years of smoking.

If you are relying on repression of your desire to smoke as the way to stop smoking, it is just a question of time before you feel a desire and start smoking again.

There are a number of techniques that help smokers to repress their desire. Most forms of acupuncture and hypnosis are attempts to do that. So, too, is aversion therapy. If the technique helps a smoker to repress effectively, then it's likely to have a good short-term success rate. Let's take a closer look at aversion techniques, as it is very likely you have been trying this approach, without necessarily realising it.

A Filthy Mess

Most people, whether they smoke or not, have some adverse thoughts about smoking. Certainly people who have never smoked often hate everything about it: all they see is that it smells foul, creates mess, and is bad for your health.

Many smokers also find smoking revolting, at least on some occasions. The morning after a party, for example, they can feel sickened physically and mentally by all the cigarettes they got through the night before. Then they won't have any desire to smoke at all, or a very minor one that can easily be ignored.

One well-known aversion technique makes use of this phenomenon by instructing the smoker to smoke rapidly and excessively, focusing on how much the smoke hurts and burns and makes you feel ill. Another technique is to deliver electric shocks as you smoke, and a slightly less drastic one is to snap a rubber band round your wrist. The idea is to create an association between smoking and pain. An aversion can also be developed simply by repeating, over and over again, how evil, filthy and useless smoking is.

In all cases, the intention is the same: to put you off wanting to smoke, and so override the desire for a cigarette. Then, whenever you think of smoking, or whenever someone offers you a cigarette, your reaction is meant to be one of disgust and revulsion.

It's one way of stopping, and for a few people it can work in the long term as well. You have probably met the kind of ex-smoker who makes a great deal of this, reiterating over and over again how smoking is dirty and repulsive and smelly and unhealthy. They are acting out their own aversion, reinforcing it by talking about it.

So what's the problem? Well, in order to work long term, the aversion has to be absolute and unequivocal. And the problem with that is that the human mind is complex and often contradictory (any human mind, not just yours!) Most people find it impossible to remain so utterly single-minded, especially when it comes to an addiction. The hung-over smoker mentioned before is thoroughly sickened, all morning, by the idea of smoking. But as the hangover fades, so does the aversion. The smoker begins to feel like smoking again and is puffing away as usual by the end of the day.

You can work very hard at developing aversive thoughts, but it is inevitable that you will also have some positive memories of smoking. An addiction means that you're attracted to whatever it is you are addicted to, and that feeling of attraction will return at some point.

It is entirely possible to be totally convinced, at one moment, that smoking is the most loathsome and foul thing on earth, and yet, moments later, to be completely enveloped in a powerful desire to smoke, believing that smoking a cigarette would be enjoyable, exciting and life-enhancing. Both these extremes co-exist in the mind of the smoker and they continue to do so after the smoker has stopped.

That feeling of attraction will return at some point.

It is, of course, entirely realistic to have adverse thoughts about smoking. That's probably what makes you want to stop smoking in the first place. The truth is that smoking does burn your throat, it does make you feel ill and it does smell foul. (By the way, if you are unwilling to acknowledge these facts at all, it's because you are terrified of feeling deprived, as Chapter 4 will explain.) It's fine to remember these things, but don't expect them to eliminate your desire to smoke. An aversion to smoking which results in repression of the addictive desire is a very temporary way of stopping.

Sooner or later, you will experience the return of your desire to smoke. It may be when you are under stress, or while relaxing on holiday. It may be when you feel miserable and alone, or when you are thoroughly enjoying yourself at a party, surrounded by friends.

If you want to stop smoking and stay stopped this time, you are much more likely to succeed if you learn to live with that reality. It isn't your aversion that will keep you from smoking, but your ability to cope with your feeling of wanting to smoke.

Repression Doesn't Work

There are more problems associated with repression, however, than the simple fact that most people can't keep it up for ever.

First of all there are the extraordinary lengths some people go to in order to reach the impossible goal of ridding themselves of their desire for a smoke. Avoiding anything that might make you want to smoke, including other smokers in both work and social situations, soon becomes an impractical and inconvenient charade. Keeping yourself occupied at all times also turns out to be impossible.

Clients of mine have told me all sorts of weird and wonderful strategies they have devised on previous desperate attempts to quit. One woman who lived in the country told me that every time she wanted to smoke, she went outside and ran as fast as she could all the way round her house, screaming loudly. Another said that for a while he tried smoking only while he was standing on his head, the theory being that by breaking down all other cues to smoke, he would only want to smoke when upside down. Because this would happen so rarely, eventually he would be free from the desire to smoke!

Needless to say, both these approaches failed, which is why these smokers ended up on my course. I should add that both have now stopped and have not smoked since. Their success this time was the result of learning a completely different attitude towards their desire to smoke.

A more serious problem with repression can be understood when you realise that the desire to smoke is an energy, a physical force not unlike emotions such as anger and grief. It is now widely accepted that chronic repression of emotions leads to physical upsets of all kinds. With stopping smoking, the effect of repressing your desire to smoke can surface in symptoms such as excess hunger, tension, loss of sleep, poor concentration and taking up other compulsive behaviours, such as shopping.

Repressive techniques don't work for most people in the long term.

Defusing the Bomb

The irony is that ex-smokers tend to feel quite confident while they are repressing their desire to smoke. It seems to them that they have their problem under control and that they have truly broken the addiction this time. It's a very common and attractive error to see the absence of addictive desire as a sign of having succeeded.

But repression is, at best, a temporary way to stop smoking. It's like sitting on a time bomb: the only question is when it will explode. And when it does, you can be smoking before you even have a chance to know what is happening. If you do not have your mind trained to deal with the desire, you might not even be able to notice it, let alone control it.

Repressive techniques will be effective for a few people, but they don't work for most people in the long term.[1]

The technique this book describes takes an entirely different approach. It is based on the fact that the desire to smoke cannot be completely and permanently eliminated. It's about learning how to face up to it, and deal with it. If you do that, you defuse the time bomb. It may seem more difficult in the beginning; but you will lose the fear of the bomb going off later on. And this time you get the opportunity to stay stopped.

Real Control

When you learn how to manage your desire to smoke, you have every chance of success in staying stopped for good. You don't fight it, you don't try to ignore it or make it go away. You remember that repression or avoidance of the desire removes the problem only temporarily; it doesn't solve it. In fact, it's only when you cope with the desire to smoke that you are really in control. The desire will diminish in time, but the first thing is to expect it. It's not a sign of weakness or impending failure: it's a perfectly normal aspect of being an ex-smoker. In fact, it is the way you become an ex-smoker.

Once you have stopped, the urge to smoke will happen less and less often. But it's not just the infrequency of desire that will keep you from smoking; it's that you will have learned how to deal with it.

You will be able to see it for what it is, separate it from whatever else is happening, and make a choice about what you want to do.

IN OTHER WORDS: GILL

Although I wanted to stop smoking, I had severe doubts that I could. When I started the course I was on about 30 a day. I enjoyed some cigarettes very much; the majority I did not and I felt uncomfortable being so tied to something that most of the time was a habit rather than a pleasure. I realised I had completely lost control over my smoking.

During the course, because of my misgivings, I think I was unconsciously resisting the technique. I frequently felt cross and couldn't believe it could possibly work. However, I followed the instructions and guidelines. The first few days were very difficult but, unlike the time I had stopped smoking before, the grim period passed within two weeks.

To me, the most important aspect of the technique was that it allowed me to feel the desire to smoke and not to feel frightened of that. This permission is, in fact, one's eventual freedom. The desire to smoke stops being something to be terrified of, to dread, and to want to suppress. Once that awful pressure comes off, one quietly stops smoking.

A year on I feel quite secure around cigarettes and other smokers. They don't bother me. I don't feel I want to boast that I've stopped smoking; I just accept and am glad that it has happened. For me it has been a 'quiet revolution' and because it has been a quiet one, I feel confident that it will last.

CHAPTER 4

Your Freedom to Smoke

Adam was but human – this explains it all. He did not want the apple for the apple's sake, he wanted it only because it was forbidden.
MARK TWAIN

It's a common myth that smokers don't have willpower, or not as much as other people. But willpower isn't something that gets handed out in finite amounts: everybody has will and the power to use it.

So why is it that some people aren't able to make good use of their will to stop smoking? The answer to this is crucial to understand. What you need to know about will is that it only works when it is freely directed. Our will is free will, and a great many smokers make the fatal mistake of believing that they surrender their free will when they stop smoking. They think that stopping smoking means losing their freedom to smoke.

Thinking this way has disastrous consequences: the misery of feeling deprived.

What You Think is What You Will Feel

The most important thing to understand about feeling deprived is that it is purely and simply the result of a particular way of thinking. And you can change the way you think.

The way of thinking that creates feelings of deprivation is to deny freedom of choice by believing, for example: 'I have to stop smoking!' and 'I can't fail this time!' It is these 'have to' and 'can't' thoughts that create feelings of deprivation. They are actually feelings of anger, resentment, loss, frustration and self-pity that spring from thinking you are denied access to something you want.

But if you think more carefully about it, you rarely are denied access to cigarettes for any length of time. The only way you could be is if you were physically locked up somewhere without any cigarettes and with no means of escape! Then you would not be free to smoke. You genuinely would not have any choice about it. But this is the only kind of situation in which it is actually true that your freedom to smoke has been lost.

If you were locked up in a cell without cigarettes, then your feelings of deprivation would be appropriate. Most smokers would get angry and stressed if they had that kind of restriction imposed on them. Most smokers would feel sorry for themselves if other people were free to smoke while they weren't.

You see, after you stop smoking, if you believe you can't smoke, your mind will react exactly as if you were locked up in a cell with no access to cigarettes.

So, if you don't remind yourself of your freedom of choice, if instead you use prohibiting, restricting words, like 'I can't smoke' or 'I mustn't smoke', then you will feel as if you are depriving yourself. And you will rebel against this just as surely as if your cigarettes had in fact been forbidden.

The feelings we call 'deprivation' are always based on the delusion that our freedom is being denied. If you make free choices, out of your own free will, it will be obvious you are not being deprived – or depriving yourself – even though you are not smoking.

'I Have to Stop' . . . but Not Today

Even while you are still smoking, you may well be thinking to yourself, 'I have to stop.' Many smokers say this to themselves every day. A common train of thought is: 'If I go on smoking, my health will deteriorate. I can't let that happen, so, I have to stop smoking.'

In fact, this is never true. When you believe that you 'have to' stop, you fail to acknowledge that you've got the freedom to continue – whether you want that freedom or not! You do, in fact, have the freedom to go on smoking and have your health deteriorate. This doesn't mean that you *will* go on smoking; it just means you've got the option of doing so.

This doesn't mean that you will go on smoking; it just means you've got the option of doing so.

If you stop smoking believing you 'have to' stop, you are telling yourself you have no choice about it. You are telling yourself that you are being forced, or forcing yourself, to stop. Then stopping smoking becomes, instead of the liberation it really is, a sentence of doom.

It feels like a sentence of doom because you feel as if you have been trapped, or that you have trapped yourself. It's no wonder smokers keep procrastinating about stopping! Many smokers live through their whole lives telling themselves that they 'have to' stop smoking – but not today.

A thought that has quite different implications is: 'I want

to stop smoking.' However, as soon as anyone gets serious about stopping, their attitude is often: 'I don't really want to stop, but I have to.' And they completely forget that stopping smoking is something they *want* to do.

When you accept that you don't ever have to, you may begin to see that, in fact, you do really want to.

Symptoms of Deprivation

Most smokers believe themselves to be deprived, to some degree, during the process of stopping smoking, but the experience can be very different for different kinds of people. This partly depends on how strongly the denial of choice is believed.

Anger and irritability are very common. Some ex-smokers will pick fights with people, become intolerant, impatient, aggressive and even rude. It can seem that their personality has completely changed since they stopped smoking.

Ex-smokers in a state of deprivation will often feel a sense of panic. They feel stressed, restless and can even get symptoms of extreme anxiety such as palpitations, sweating and trembling. They will feel tense as well, clenching muscles in the jaw, neck, shoulders and hands.

Some feel martyred and resentful about having stopped. All the fun has gone out of their lives. They may become profoundly depressed, withdrawn and apathetic, even to the point of thinking that a life without smoking may not be worth living. There is often a deep sense of self-pity and it is not unusual to start envying other people who are still smoking. They think, 'Poor me, lucky them.'

When people feel deprived, they often see stopping smoking as a great loss. Tears are shed, as if something wonderful has been taken away from them, against their will. They feel like victims. It feels like there's a huge void in their life that won't ever be filled.

At this stage, your past life as a smoker can begin to look like 'the good old days'. You become obsessed with smoking, and begin to figure out ways to justify going back to it. Perhaps you start an argument with someone (especially a person who has been pushing you to stop), or you stage some kind of drama so that you have a good excuse to smoke. Or you make do with a not-so-good excuse.

While you have a sense of deprivation your desire to smoke won't diminish. It becomes exaggerated, more intense, and you can still be yearning for a smoke for hours at a time, months after stopping – if you can keep yourself from smoking for that long.

Perhaps the most undermining effect of this state of deprivation is that you completely lose sight of your motivation to stay stopped. Maybe when you were smoking, you were longing to stop. You were sick of smoking, desperately wanting to get it out of your life for ever. So you stopped, but now, instead of feeling joy and relief, you feel as if you are being punished – even tortured! You don't see anything good at all about not smoking. Life without smoking looks dull and boring. And then you really can't remember one reason why you ever thought of giving up such a fabulous pastime!

If you allow a state of deprivation to persist, it's going to be virtually impossible for you to stay stopped.

Feeling deprived makes stopping smoking dramatic and unbearable, and blows everything up out of all proportion. One person may feel a bit light-headed and disorientated for the first day after they've stopped, but they take that in their stride. Someone experiencing deprivation will over-react to that by thinking they are losing their mind.

If you allow a state of deprivation to persist, it's going to be virtually impossible for you to stay stopped: *it's very difficult to stay motivated to keep on depriving yourself!*

Difficult Circumstances

There are certain circumstances that make it more likely for someone to deny their freedom of choice, and experience deprivation as a consequence. If one of the following situations applies to you, however, it doesn't mean you will be unable to stop smoking. It means you are likely to feel deprived at first. The more effort you put into developing a genuine sense of choice, the faster you'll overcome this difficulty.

- Serious health fears. Possibly the most common and strongest sense of deprivation is found in smokers who are deeply concerned about the state of their health. If you have become really frightened by symptoms such as angina, severe coughing or gasping for breath, you can become too frightened to even consider the possibility that you could continue to smoke. You may even have had a doctor tell you, in no uncertain terms, that you 'have to' stop.

  The irony is that if you don't change your thinking you are likely to end up smoking, despite your best intentions and efforts to stop. If left uncorrected, the strength of your belief that you have no choice creates such a powerful sense of deprivation that staying stopped becomes extraordinarily difficult.

- Illness of a relative or friend. If you ever have witnessed a serious illness and/or death from a smoking-related disease, you will almost certainly have formed a strong belief that you simply 'can't' let that happen to you.
- Specific health problems. You might have a particular health problem that, although not caused by smoking, will contribute to the belief that you aren't free to smoke. People with diabetes or asthma often feel especially pressured to stop by their condition. You might have been born with a particular weakness of the lungs or heart.
- Pressure from other people. As a smoker, you may be told incessantly that you 'have to' stop smoking, or that you 'can't smoke' in certain situations. Loved ones may threaten to leave you, or may try to strike bargains aimed at pressuring you to stop. Everywhere you go, it seems that people are telling you that you 'can't smoke' any more. (Or 'must not', 'should not' or 'ought not', which give rise to the same feelings.) If you stop smoking primarily because someone else has asked or told you to, it can feel as if you have no choice in the matter yourself, and this can create an intolerable state of deprivation.
- Obligation. Stopping smoking because of a sense of obligation to others is another way in which people create feelings of deprivation. Parents may feel obliged to stop because of the effect of their smoking on their children, both in the sense of being bad role models and because of the dangers of passive smoking.
- Pregnancy. Obviously the obligation to an unborn child can create a powerful belief that you 'have to' stop smoking. And the sense of deprivation that arises from this can make it very difficult to do.

It's not that pregnant women don't have good reasons to stop smoking; they certainly do. The point is that there is a crucial difference between having good reasons to stop and thinking that your free will has been taken away.

- Role models and closet smokers. You might work in a job that creates a particular kind of pressure to stop smoking. You may believe, because of your profession, that you should set a good example for others, and should not be seen to be a smoker.

  You may even hide the fact that you smoke and become a closet (secret) smoker. Nicotine gum can be a way for someone to hide their smoking, but a sense of deprivation keeps the addiction fuelled. This may be particularly true among people in health professions, and the clergy.

  Another kind of closet smoker hides their smoking because they are so obviously ill from it, and the tremendous guilt they feel, if not dealt with in the correct way, is sure to lead to a very strong sense of deprivation whenever they make an attempt to stop smoking.
- Your upbringing. If you had authoritarian (or very permissive) parents it's likely you were not taught how to make your own choices about anything. All children need some encouragement to consider choosing between delayed and instant gratification, and unfortunately many never get to learn this. If you were simply told that smoking is a sin and you must never do it, it's understandable that you regard it as forbidden. Stopping smoking, even much later on in life, can still be seen as a capitulation to the order 'thou shalt not smoke', resulting in a strong sense of deprivation.

'Can't, Must, Got to, Have to'

A great many people see all kinds of things in life in terms of things that they 'have to' or 'can't' do, so stopping smoking becomes just one more thing they approach with this attitude.

'Can't' and 'have to' are frequently misused in everyday thought and speech. For example, you might say: 'I can't have dinner with you tonight.' This, of course, does not usually mean that you're physically incapable or forbidden. It simply means you have another engagement that you prefer to keep.

Often, this choice of words doesn't create much of a problem. In fact, many people get lots of things accomplished by believing that they have no choice but to do them. When it comes to stopping smoking, however, your choice of words – and therefore the way you think – can make the difference between failure and success because of the intolerable problem of feeling deprived.

If you are the sort of person who says 'I have to' and 'I can't' a lot, you will need to work hard to alter your way of thinking. And if you do this with smoking, the overall benefit can affect many other areas of your life as well. Freedom feels good!

Own Your Choices and You Take Control

Feeling deprived indicates that you are not taking full responsibility for your own actions. If you really are locked up without cigarettes, your jailer is responsible for the fact that you are not smoking – not you.

It's an error we are all susceptible to, because in each of us there remains the little child we once were, the record in our memories of a time when we really weren't responsible for ourselves. When you stop smoking, by telling yourself 'You are not allowed to smoke!' the child in you becomes actively rebellious.

Becoming psychologically responsible is something we all do by degrees. It is the process of coming to recognise that you are the creator of what you think, feel and do. And it is you and you alone who determines whether you smoke or not!

You might be the kind of person who has difficulty in doing that because you have a strong tendency to blame others, refusing to see your own part in any of the situations in your life. Whether you are smoking or stopping smoking, you see it as just one more thing that makes you a victim of circumstance.

So when you stop smoking, you subconsciously blame others and project your anger on to the people around you – family, friends or complete strangers.

Some end up believing they are really very angry people and that smoking is the only thing that keeps their anger under wraps. It certainly can seem that way if you don't understand what's really going on.

If this seems to apply to you, all you need to do is remember that stopping smoking is your choice, and that nobody else has done this to you. You may feel angry and resentful when you stop, but it's because you have forgotten about your freedom of choice. All you need to do is remind yourself.

By the way, if you are trying to stop smoking purely because of someone else, my advice to you is: don't.

Sacrifice and Reward

When you think you can't smoke, smoking becomes forbidden fruit, and, as everybody knows, that's always the sweetest. In order to compensate for this sense of sacrifice, you will feel a great need to reward yourself. The rewards can take the form of buying extravagant presents for yourself or eating extra, especially 'forbidden' foods, such as chocolate.

You can also think that you ought to be rewarded in some way by your family and friends and can get very upset with them for not being especially nice to you when you've stopped smoking. This is particularly likely if you have stopped smoking to please them.

If you approach stopping as a choice rather than as a deprivation, you will be able to see that not smoking is its own reward. Your health will improve and you will feel proud of yourself and more in control of your life. And if being an ex-smoker isn't a preferable, more rewarding way of life for you, then you can always go back to being a smoker! If you choose that it may, of course, cost you your health, and it's very likely that you will increasingly regret your dependence on smoking. But either way, it is simply your choice about how you want to live your life. Living your life as a smoker has its consequences. But smoking is not forbidden! You are allowed to be a smoker. You always have permission to smoke – whether you actually do it or not.

If you have stopped smoking in the past and you felt deprived, then when you did finally smoke, it probably seemed like a rewarding thing to do. You may have experienced a mixture of feelings: disappointment at your failure, but also a great sense of release. This is because smoking a cigarette seems to release you from that imaginary cell of your deprivation. In as much as it relieves the symptoms of the 'deprivation', it will cheer you up, calm you down, please and reward you. This is why it's so important to overcome your beliefs about being deprived. If you don't, you may end up reinforcing your sense of dependency on cigarettes.

Rebellion

If it seems to you that stopping smoking has locked you up in that cell of deprivation, smoking a cigarette will be your key to freedom. Many smokers find themselves stuck with smoking, unable to stop even for the briefest time, purely in order to maintain a sense of freedom. It's a crazy trap.

A rebellion always means that a restriction has been imposed. You cannot rebel if you are already free.

You can tell when 'rebellious' smokers are anticipating feeling deprived because they increase the amount they are smoking whenever they get serious about stopping, or are told to stop by a doctor. They are making sure that they don't feel trapped and deprived even before they stop smoking! These are the people who believe they 'have to' stop, and are already rebelling against that imagined restriction.

Many smokers make attempts to stop smoking, only to feel deprived because of their denial of choice, and then go back to smoking in order to prove, once again, that they are free to smoke: 'Nobody can tell me what to do! I can smoke and I will! I'll show them!'

A rebellion always means that a restriction has been imposed. You cannot rebel if you are already free.

Feeling Free

The truth is that you are free to be a smoker. There will be consequences for you should you take that path. But these consequences, however terrifying, do not take away your freedom to smoke. They are the consequences you get if you exercise that freedom by smoking.

This is your life, and you are free to live it as a smoker if that is your choice. You can smoke. You can go on smoking. You can smoke even more each day than you do now. You can smoke every day of your life and never stop.

I'm not encouraging you to do that: living your life as a smoker will cost you dearly. It will cost you your health, your money and your self-esteem. It may also cost you jobs, relationships and even years of your life.

What I'm encouraging you to do is to find a way to stop smoking without feeling deprived, so that you will be able to stay stopped and feel happy about that. And the way to do that is to understand – and really believe – that stopping smoking doesn't limit your freedom to smoke, in any way.

The most important thing to know about stopping smoking is: you don't have to do it. Ever!

Does this sound like a dangerous way of thinking? It's very possible that you are afraid to tell yourself you are free to be a smoker. The fear, of course, is that if you give yourself that option of smoking, you will actually take it. So you try to eliminate it by convincing yourself you have no choice but to stop and stay stopped. And that's exactly how you create the misery of feeling deprived.

Overcoming Deprivation

If you are reading this as a smoker, the fact that you're free to smoke might seem rather obvious. Here you are, lighting up cigarettes and smoking them. Of course you can do that. It's after you have made an attempt to stop that your choice to go back to smoking can seem to have been surrendered.

The work involved in stopping smoking is in coming to understand that you have the freedom to return to smoking – even though you are not exercising that freedom by smoking.

The chances are that you have a deep-seated belief that you have been developing for many years, even decades. And it takes some time and effort to turn this false way of thinking around.

A recent client of mine, Susan, is typical of someone working through a substantial problem with deprivation. When she first stopped smoking she got very angry, then lethargic and apathetic. When I spoke to her a week later she was feeling very deprived, yearning to smoke for hours on end, even though she was genuinely horrified by the thought of going back to smoking. Understandably, she said that she didn't feel very confident at all. She told me that she couldn't smoke. Her (false) logic was that if she wanted to stay off smoking, then she didn't have the option of smoking. 'If I want to live,' she said, 'then I can't smoke.' 'Not true,' I told her. 'You want to live; true. Smoking will kill you; that is possible. But the truth is that you still have the option of doing that. It's a freedom you have, whether you want it or not. It's a fact of life.'

I wasn't encouraging her to smoke, I was encouraging her to acknowledge that the choice to smoke exists, so that she wouldn't think she was being deprived. When she turned this thinking around she felt much more positive and in control, and found staying stopped much easier.

Her background explains the trouble she was having coming to terms with the concept of free choice. Her parents were both heavy smokers. While they smoked and smoked every day, they always told her, over and over again, that she 'must never become a smoker'. They were both very ill from smoking, and understandably wanted a better life for their daughter. Susan started smoking when she was 16 and you can imagine the reaction when her parents found out. There was much screaming and yelling, and again she was told that she was not allowed to smoke, that she 'had to stop'.

Once, a few years ago, she stopped smoking after a visit to a hypnotist, but she had just repressed her desire, and was back smoking after two weeks. She didn't even see the issue of choice and deprivation until she came to my course, after 30 years of smoking, simultaneously believing she just wasn't allowed to smoke.

When she reminds herself that she does, in fact, have the freedom to smoke, not smoking becomes easier and far more positive. Her desire to smoke is significantly more tolerable, when before it was 'like a scream through my body'. Knowing she has a choice provided the key.

She goes through periods of forgetting her freedom, but then she will remember it again, eventually shifting her thinking enough so that her choices are real to her.

Sometimes it does take a while for the penny to drop, and this is what causes the initial difficulty in stopping smoking. It's important to keep on repeating to yourself that you are totally free to be a smoker. You may understand that you have the choice to smoke, but only on a relatively superficial level. You see the logic, but inside you are still fighting against the belief that you are not free at all. It takes a while for your thinking to change on every level.

Many people feel the effects of thinking they are deprived, but are not aware of the thinking that is causing them. In fact, most people aren't even aware that it is thinking that is causing them at all.

Often a client who has been feeling deprived for a week or two will say to me, 'When will it get better?' 'When you change the way you are thinking,' I reply. A common mistake is to believe that the sense of deprivation is caused by something physical, like a flu virus, and must be patiently tolerated until it runs its course. I have seen the transformation in so many people, though, who have made that all-important shift in their thinking and instantly stopped feeling deprived!

- If you feel angry, remind yourself that nobody is making you do this and that you have not trapped yourself: you are free to return to smoking, whether you actually do that or not. It's up to you.
- If you feel grief, remember that you have not lost anything; smoking is completely available to you.
- If you forget your motivation, remember that you are not locked into one irrevocable decision: you can become a smoker again. Consider that option carefully and honestly, and if there's anything you like about not smoking, it will become obvious.

Stopping smoking doesn't have to feel like a restriction and a tragedy: it can be a liberation and a genuine reward. But you will only experience it that way while you really understand you have still got the freedom to be a smoker if you so choose.

That choice doesn't exist only at the time you stop. A return to smoking continues to be an alternative for the rest of your life, and this can be difficult to accept, especially if you have a strong fear of failure. How to enjoy your continued freedom to smoke – and not deny it or fear it – is what we will be looking at next.

IN OTHER WORDS: RUTH

I began smoking when I was about eight, but did not take it up seriously until I was 14 or 15. My intake rose steadily until in my early forties I was smoking around 80 cigarettes a day. If I happened to stay up late, as I quite often did, I could go up to 120.

I tried to stop on a number of occasions. My main reason for wanting to stop was self-disgust at my utter dependence and the fact that they really had come to dominate my life. I fretted about not being able to smoke on the tube or in the houses of those who objected.

What was most helpful in the Full Stop course was the removal of that sense of mental deprivation that essentially wrecked every previous attempt of mine to stop smoking. The training of my subconscious to grasp that I wasn't being prevented from smoking, but was utterly free to do so at any time, was what made a crucial difference.

The best thing about not smoking is the sense of freedom. I encourage friends of mine to give up according to this method, but I don't nag. One of the other great virtues of the course was that it didn't turn me into one of those awful converts who go around condemning smokers. I am untroubled by having smokers around me. My house is full of ashtrays, I don't mind the smell even of stale smoke, and active smoke I quite enjoy.

CHAPTER 5

Choosing for Now

Nothing ever happened in the past; it happened in the Now. Nothing will ever happen in the future; it will happen in the Now.
ECKHART TOLLE, *THE POWER OF NOW*

Many people who have attended my course tell me, much later on, that they never expected to succeed. The chances are they had tried to stop many times before, both on their own and with other kinds of help, and had failed over and over again. It's probable that you also, to a greater or lesser extent, have a conviction that even if you stop, you will not be able to stay stopped for very long. It's a common and understandable concern to have. The problem, however, is not with your expectation of failure, but with the way you try to cope with it.

To begin with, you may cope with it by not making any attempt at all to stop smoking: if you don't try, you won't fail! You may tell yourself you are waiting until you feel more motivated, because then, you think, you will be more likely to succeed. However, the motivation you are likely to be waiting for is a threat to your health: most smokers justify their smoking by reasoning that if anything serious really did happen, then of course they would stop.

But bad health doesn't remove your concerns about failure, *it increases them.* I have talked to a great many smokers who find themselves stuck between the devil and the deep blue sea: fearing not trying to stop because smoking is causing serious illness, and fearing making an attempt that fails.

Sooner or later, though, your fears push you into trying to stop. You make a solemn vow never to smoke again. You reason that in order to stop smoking and successfully stay stopped, you must make a commitment that, once made, you are bound to keep. It's a final decision, made once and for all, and the possibility of smoking again is not to be considered.

The Commitment Trap

The irony is that it is precisely this way of thinking that keeps so many smokers from even attempting to stop. Or, even if they do, it is absolutely bound to make them feel such deprivation that it becomes unbearable to keep to their commitment! Making a commitment never to smoke again is simply denying your freedom to smoke. And as you know from the last chapter, denying your freedom to smoke means that you will feel deprived. The problem, however, is that for many people the possibility of failure is so awful they think it's safer to think in terms of making one choice to quit smoking that will have to last for ever.

Of course, if you really could eliminate your freedom to return to smoking, you would indeed be secure. If you really were locked up for ever in a cell with no cigarettes, you would definitely be successful at stopping smoking! But, assuming you live in a free world with access to cigarettes, this sense of security is an extremely dangerous illusion.

This explains why it is that some smokers can appear to be so very motivated to stop, yet fail over and over again. The more desperate they are to stop smoking, the more they throw themselves into a commitment to stop for ever, and the more trapped and deprived they end up feeling. So, after a brief and agonising period of time, they break down and smoke, only to feel even more desperate the next time they try to stop. It's a vicious circle! And, unless you are aware of the attitude you are taking, you may create this very situation for yourself.

Overcome your fear of failure without denying your freedom to fail.

As with all the difficulties that smokers create in their attempts to stop, there is a way to change your thinking so it becomes much more positive, realistic and attainable. If you really want to stay stopped this time, you need to overcome your fear of failure without denying your freedom to fail. *And the way to do that is to choose to stop smoking only for the present time.*

Now, Now, and Now . . .

If you make a choice to stop smoking, how long does that choice last? You might want it to last for at least a day. You might want it to last for a few days. But life doesn't work that way.

The truth is that you can only make a choice as to whether you smoke or not when you actually make it, right in that moment, in the here and now. If you make a choice to stop smoking at 12.30, then even before 12.31 you have a whole new choice to make. Because you've got free will, you could choose to smoke at 12.31! Or you could make another choice not to smoke.

When you stop smoking, you don't start out by making a commitment to never smoke again. You start out by making a choice not to smoke only for that moment. And you bear in mind that you will be making many more choices as you 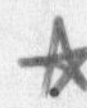 go along.

At first, this may sound unbearable, even impossible. It seems a lot easier to make one resolution and convince yourself that you 'have to' stick to it. But remember, in fact, this is a much more difficult route. Once you have truly accepted this principle, making choices only for the present time will become simple, obvious, more positive and *much easier*. Remember also that the desire to smoke, and therefore the process of making choices, becomes much less frequent as time goes on.

When you stop smoking by declaring 'I've smoked my last cigarette – I'll never smoke again!' you deny your freedom to smoke, and put yourself straight into the cell of deprivation. Even if you predict that you won't smoke for the next hour, then for that hour you are going to feel deprived.

By all means have the goal of staying stopped. By all means have a clear intention not to smoke again. But as you do this, remember that you can only reach that goal by making real choices in the here and now. This means you acknowledge that you have the option of going back to smoking and there's always the possibility that you could do that. Knowing this makes the crucial difference between feeling miserably deprived and feeling free and in control.

Loss and Grief

Smokers often describe their experience of stopping as a process of grieving. They see their cigarettes as companions with whom they had a kind of relationship for a major part of their lives. When smokers 'give up' this relationship, they often say they are mourning a great loss, the passing on of these 'friends'.

There are, however, crucial distinctions. First of all, cigarettes aren't your friends, any more than a bottle of booze is a friend to an alcoholic or a syringe to a heroin addict. This is nothing but a delusion of drug addiction.

Even more significant, though, is that you don't lose these 'friends' when you stop smoking. The sense of loss comes from thinking you'll never smoke again. When someone dies, they are gone for ever. That's why you grieve: you will never see them again. It's final and you have absolutely no choice in the matter.

When you make choices in the present time, you keep in sight the fact that you have the freedom to return to smoking at any point. There is always the possibility that you could go back to smoking. And there is always the possibility that you could end up stuck with it – *smoking every day for the rest of your life.*

If you really take that fact in, you'll know there is no need to grieve. You will be aware, of course, that you are not smoking, but there is a big difference between noticing that you've stopped and feeling as if you've lost something you can never get back again.

At first, staying stopped can be a bit of a balancing act, like walking along the edge of a cliff, knowing that you could make one false move and end it all. Instead of pretending that the cliff doesn't exist, what works is to master walking along this edge.

Pressure from Others

During the first couple of weeks after you have stopped, it's especially helpful to remember about choosing for now when you talk to others about your smoking. If you have taken my advice and kept the whole thing quiet, it might be a while before they catch on to what you are doing. As you can probably now see, the longer you keep quiet about having stopped, the better.

Sooner or later, though, someone will notice that you haven't been smoking and they might ask you directly if you've stopped. It's going to be best for you to say something that doesn't make you feel as though you've made a permanent commitment. Say something like: 'Well, I'm cutting down, I don't know if I'll stop,' or 'I might 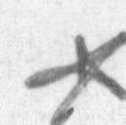 have one later.' It doesn't matter what they think. What matters is that you have kept in touch with your choices. So far, so good. You haven't locked yourself into one, irrevocable decision.

If you go around telling everybody you've stopped smoking, you can create a stronger sense of being trapped into not smoking, which is disastrous for your motivation. Their pressure on you to stay stopped will act to enhance your sense of deprivation, and that's the very last thing you need. Other people can put the pressure on in the most innocent ways, even by saying things like: 'Good for you!' or 'Keep it up!' If you are feeling deprived, you might want to hit them! It's also likely you'll find yourself close to lighting up a cigarette. It's just as if they are telling you that you can't ever smoke again, so all you want to do is rebel to assert your freedom.

Margaret, a woman in her fifties who had smoked for over 40 years, told me about a conversation she had with her father a few weeks after she had attended a course with me. Her father took her hand and, with tears in his eyes, thanked her sincerely for having stopped smoking, saying that he was immensely proud of what she had done.

Margaret told me that although she knew he was expressing his love for her, and that his acknowledgement was very much appreciated, she felt a surge of rebellion well up inside her as he spoke. She thanked him for his concern, and privately reminded herself that she was still free to go back to smoking. She continues to make free choices not to smoke, just for now, based on what she wants for herself.

Other clients have had similar difficult reactions, suddenly feeling obliged to stay stopped as a result of gifts – a piece of jewellery or a bunch of flowers – given as a reward for stopping.

I'll Worry About It When I Get There

There's another kind of problem that comes from trying to make choices in the future. It's common when you first stop smoking to get worried about particular activities or events, wondering if you will actually be able to handle them without smoking.

You might be anxious about a party or an especially demanding work project. It might be meeting that old friend with whom you used to chain-smoke and talk for hours. Or it might be a familiar activity, like talking on the phone or driving long distances, where you have developed an especially strong connection with smoking. Whatever it is, you can bet there will be something that you'll become concerned about after you have stopped.

You might try to project yourself into the future and imagine yourself doing these things without smoking. This will not be helpful. It's quite possible that your mind does not have a picture of you doing these things without smoking, so it cannot deal with them at all. You have no experience, no memory to refer to.

You can create a tremendous amount of anxiety because you are sure you will never make it through this situation without smoking. Since you can't imagine it, having never done it, the anxiety keeps building up. If you don't overcome your anxiety, the next step is for you to smoke because you are sure that you will end up doing that at some point anyway.

But it's not the situation that causes you to smoke – it's your anxiety about the future situation. It's your fear of failure that leads you to fail.

I'm not going to suggest that you should never think about the future, because that's impossible. It would be ridiculous to pretend that you will never think at all about certain situations, and whether or not you'll smoke. But if you start to worry and get anxious about them, simply remind yourself that you can only choose whether or not you smoke in present time. You have no way of knowing how you will handle a situation in the future. You can never know whether or not you will smoke at the party on Saturday night until you are there, making your choices.

The key to success is being willing to not know for sure. Of course, it would be comforting to have a guarantee that you won't fail, but the fact is, there is always a risk, and that's just the way life is. You might smoke again and you might not. All you can do is choose for now not to smoke and hope you continue to do that.

By all means anticipate a strong desire to smoke when you are in a particular situation: just remember that you can only manage that desire at the time you are experiencing it.

You can only smoke in the present time. And you can

only choose not to smoke in the present time. Accept that you are not able to predict which choice you'll make in the future. When you deal with not smoking in the here and now, you put yourself in a position of control.

So Far, So Good

The chances are that you won't feel confident at first. If you have been smoking, daily, for many years, not smoking will quite possibly feel very strange at first, even unnatural. But the longer you stay off and the more situations you handle without smoking, the more confident you become. Confidence is something you acquire, gradually.

The techniques described in Part Two of this book are very effective. The more effort you put into working with them, the more confident you will become not only that they work, but that you are capable of using them. You learn to trust yourself that you will continue to use them, no matter what is going on in your life. This is something you can only find out for yourself as you go along. It's difficult to feel sure of it ahead of time.

When you deal with not smoking in the here and now, you put yourself in a position of control.

Many smokers make the mistake of putting off stopping smoking because they are waiting to feel confident. They want to wait until they are sure they will succeed before making an attempt to stop. They might be waiting for a very long time.

Don't wait for your fear of failure to go away. Stopping smoking will always be somewhat frightening, *because you never know how it will turn out.*

It's much, much less frightening if you just do it moment by moment. So far, so good, and wait and see what happens.

One client, Richard, says that he doesn't even call himself an ex-smoker because it sounds too final. He says that he is a smoker who just isn't smoking right now. He's been saying that for well over a year, so far.

Choosing for now keeps you in reality. But what happens if, after perhaps a whole year of making choices not to smoke, you then make a choice to smoke? If you have the freedom to smoke, shouldn't you exercise it at least once in a while? This is the subject of our next chapter.

IN OTHER WORDS: DEE

I don't think I ever believed I would stop smoking. I had been a smoker for 26 years. I smoked 20 to 30 a day – or 40 if life was more exciting, conversation was intense, or during panic situations. I loved my cigarette breaks and the social side that accompanied them.

The course gave me the tools to fight my battle: staying in the present time helped stop panic about even the next 10 minutes. I worked hard at stopping smoking, and every time I talked myself through a desire to smoke and gave myself the choices, I felt stronger, more proud of myself and totally surprised that I was doing it. I still am. I still have the original cigarettes in my desk with access to more if I want, but I have not had so much as one puff since I stopped two and a half years ago. And, because I don't feel that I am depriving myself of anything, I have not joined the angry mob of ex-smokers.

I was amazed to find myself having a desire to smoke recently: I went through my 'talk' and made my choice to accept the desire. I feel I have been empowered by the course and that I have given myself a huge gift by stopping smoking.

CHAPTER 6

One More Puff

The dance of the last cigarette which began when I was twenty has not reached its last figure yet . . . I may as well say that for some time past I have been smoking a great many cigarettes and have given up calling them the last.

ITALO SVEVO, *CONFESSIONS OF ZENO*

Smoking is not just a bad habit, it's a drug addiction. I'm not saying this to make you feel guilty, but to help you deal with the facts. All addictions are surrounded and supported by a collection of powerful lies, or delusions. Taking control is the process of identifying those lies and discovering the truth.

Frequently, people in the process of stopping smoking say that there are two opposing voices, like two completely different people, inside their head, arguing. Of course, you are only one, whole person: the other voice is that of the addiction you have created over the years. Some people say it's the Devil talking. This argument is part of the process of stopping smoking, and this book provides you with every bit of information you need to work through the argument and resolve this conflict.

You could think of it as a game. Any time you stop smoking, the game is that the addiction tries to figure out how to get you to go back to smoking. It will be marvellously creative and have you convinced of the most ridiculous things. You will be able to see through some of the deceptions very clearly, and maybe even laugh at them. Others may be more difficult.

Any time you stop smoking, the game is that the addiction tries to figure out how to get you to go back to smoking.

The most common, compelling and persistent of all the deceptions is the idea that, at some point, you will be able to smoke one or two cigarettes without having to return to an uncontrollable daily dependency. If you believe this to be true, it's probably the most convincing excuse to smoke there is. After all, *one* cigarette isn't going to kill you: it's 'simply not a problem'.

Of course, there are a few – just a very few – people who only smoke occasionally, which could be what makes you think it is possible. But the odds are against you.[1]

So many people go back to smoking as a direct result of this mistake. Some people even make this mistake over and over again, never learning from their past experience! It looks like such a great solution, the smoker's dream of only smoking sometimes: just at parties, or just for a day or two to help you through something difficult.

The 'something difficult' can even be withdrawal itself, which is the craziest justification of them all. Yes, smoking will certainly help ease your withdrawal symptoms, but then you will be smoking again.

When your addiction has convinced you that just one more cigarette is all you will ever want again, then you are being seriously conned.

All or Nothing

First of all, look at your own experience of smoking by estimating the total number of cigarettes you have ever smoked. You may not want to do this, but it's very powerful information. If you have smoked 20 a day for only a year, then you have already smoked about 7,300 cigarettes. If you've been at it for 10 years, you've smoked 73,000. Thirty a day for 10 years is almost 110,000 cigarettes.

Do you really think that one cigarette is all you will ever want? You do tend to smoke them one at a time, but each one is just a part of a way of life.

When you smoke, you integrate smoking into your life and you live the life of a smoker. You smoke day in, day out, year in, year out, no matter what. You smoke when you are happy and when you are sad. You smoke when you are busy and when you are bored. You smoke when you are hungry and when you are full. You smoke when you are under stress and when you are relaxing.

Of course, different people smoke different amounts; one person may smoke 20 a day and another 60. You know what kind of a smoker you are, and how much you usually smoke. That amount, whatever it is for you, is what you will be choosing to return to any time you choose to smoke. The cigarette that is just one more is really the first of thousands more.

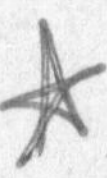

According to the *British Journal of Addiction* (1990): 'Over ninety per cent of teenagers who smoke three to four cigarettes are trapped into a career of regular smoking which typically lasts for some thirty to forty years.' If three or four cigarettes got you hooked in the first place, what are the chances of smoking just a few once the addiction has already been established?

The truth is that you are an addicted smoker, and addiction means being out of control. It is simply impossible for nicotine to become something that isn't addictive.

Resenting yourself for having become an addicted smoker won't help you at all. It is much better to admit that you did it, without blame. In fact, the more you forgive yourself for having started smoking, the more likely it is that you will stop and stay stopped. Just like millions of other people, you got conned by the same lies. It doesn't mean you are bad or stupid. It just means you are human.

This is one thing that makes smoking so different from most other drug addictions: the most stable and well-adjusted people can become totally hooked. The mistake is to refuse to believe that you have become addicted to what is arguably the most powerful addiction of them all.

I've Slipped a Bit

Eventually most smokers reluctantly come to admit that they are incapable of smoking in a controlled way. They know from their own experience that when they smoke, it's all day, every day. But another deception that smokers live with is that this way of life won't continue for long.

It's very likely that when you started smoking, you didn't think you would continue to smoke for as long as you have. You probably didn't think much about it at all, or if you did, you just thought that you'd stop some time soon – not now, of course, but before too long. Few smokers start out by intending to go on smoking every day for the rest of their lives.[2]

There is a common myth that the more times you try to stop smoking, the more likely it is that you will succeed. Repeated failures can be part of a learning process, but they can also lead to a profound sense of hopelessness about ever being able to successfully stay stopped for good.

If you think success next time will be that much more likely, remember that you also run the risk of not stopping again – *ever*. It's a possibility that very few smokers want to acknowledge. You might stop again, *but what if you don't?*

You don't have to learn everything the hard way. You don't have to get run over by a car in order to learn how to stop and look before you cross a road.

When you have stopped smoking and are considering the question of smoking again, consider this: if I choose to smoke, I will return to smoking and it's possible that I will continue to smoke every day for the rest of my life.

So is there Really a Choice?

Many people think that not being able to smoke the odd cigarette is in direct contradiction to having the freedom to smoke. Admitting that smoking one cigarette, even just lighting one up, will reignite the addiction leads many ex-smokers to conclude that they 'can't smoke ever again'.

So, once more, the ex-smoker creates feelings of deprivation. And, once more, they are caused by an error in thinking. *The choice to smoke is an all-or-nothing choice, but it's still a choice.* It's a choice to return to addictive, compulsive behaviour and run the risk of never being able to control it again. But it's still a real alternative, and a freedom that you always have.

The choice you do not have is to smoke occasionally, in a controlled, non-addictive way.

If you don't recognise that you really are free to return to smoking any time, then you might be tempted to prove that you're free by actually going ahead and doing it. 'I'll just have one' or 'I'll just smoke for a bit and stop again later' is your way out; your way of justifying smoking.

Often it is something that is done on the spur of the moment, 'without really thinking'. Many people say that if they had stopped and thought about it for a moment, then of course they would not have smoked.

That is precisely why it is so important to acknowledge the significance of lighting up a cigarette again, after you have stopped. As one of my clients explained: 'There are micro-seconds between thought and ignition, and it's only by forcing yourself into that gap that you can stop yourself from smoking.'

If, in the back of your mind, you still think that a little bit of smoking is a minor problem you can handle later, then lighting up will be a relatively easy thing to do, especially when you've got some kind of crisis as an excuse.

It's like the difference between holding a toy gun in your hands and picking up one that is real, and loaded. Cigarettes are like a real, loaded gun, and it is both helpful and appropriate to treat them with the same degree of respect for the power they possess.

How, then, should you handle the problem of 'passive smoking'? If you find yourself in a very smoky environment, you can inhale the equivalent of a couple of cigarettes and have nicotine in your blood stream. But this does not mean you will go back to smoking, as long as you have not made a choice to smoke. You may or may not experience a desire to smoke in the company of smokers, but this has no connection with passive smoking.

Once again, it's not the presence or absence of nicotine in your body, but what is going on in your mind, that can lead you to smoke. It's your mind, not your body chemistry, that will get you back smoking once you have lit a cigarette – even if you don't inhale it! This is why.

I'll Smoke One Now and Choose Not To Later

It can seem so logical: since choices last only for the moment, then after you smoke one, with your next choice you can decide not to smoke again. The trouble with this deception is that your choices aren't *equal*. You are addicted to smoking, and never become addicted to not smoking. *Your choice to smoke is your choice to return to a powerful addiction.*

Once you have smoked one cigarette, or even just part of one, you might react in a number of different ways. First of all, you might enjoy it and you might not. That really doesn't make any difference: you are just as likely to relapse if you hated your first puff.

The most common reactions are either to decide that you have failed completely and immediately go back to regular smoking – or become confident that you got away with it. Then you smoke again precisely because you believe you can get away with it.

Your return to smoking can be very gradual, even taking months, but you are at the thin end of the full-time smoking wedge.

The fewer you smoke, the better. Why get serious about stopping again when you're only smoking one or two a week? Or even one or two a day? Or five a day?

Your return to smoking can be very gradual, even taking months, but you are at the thin end of the full-time smoking wedge. During this period, it seems that you have found a way to control your smoking. The longer you keep it up, the more convincing it looks. But all that time you've kept your addiction fuelled – burning on the back of the stove – until finally it creeps back up to your usual level of daily smoking.

This deception is even more believable because of other people you probably know who do seem to keep smoking under control. The chances are that you know at least one person who smokes only sometimes, and this can seem to invalidate all the arguments about how addictive smoking is. How is it that some people can control how much they smoke, only smoking one or two at parties, for example?

There are a number of explanations. One is that they are not being completely truthful; it is common to lie to both oneself and others about any addiction. Most smokers feel guilty about smoking and their automatic defence is: 'Well, I'm not really a smoker, you know, I just have an occasional one or two at parties.' Many smokers have told me that they hide the fact that they smoke or how much they smoke.

Another possibility is that the occasional smoker is simply a relapsed ex-smoker on his way back, slowly, to regular smoking. They say that they only smoke one or two a day, and at that time it is true. But run into them a few months later and you meet a 20-a-day relapsed smoker. For most smokers it takes real effort to keep smoking under control, and they aren't able to keep it up for very long.

There are people, however, who really can control their smoking. There is a small minority of people who smoke, but simply don't ever get addicted. They really do just smoke one at Christmas. You could be one of those people, but the chances are that you are not. Otherwise, what started you on this book?

We can only guess at why those few don't get hooked. One thing to be sure of is that, for one reason or another, they don't develop the ways of thinking that create feelings of deprivation. Whether they smoke or not is not a big issue: it just doesn't matter all that much. Be assured that once it has become an issue, it will continue to be one. For the vast majority of smokers, smoking is simply not a take-it-or-leave-it kind of thing.

Good Excuses

Does it make any difference if you've got a good excuse to take that first puff? In other areas of your life, it can make all the difference. If you miss a date with a friend or an important business meeting a genuine excuse can make the difference as to whether or not you lose the friend or the job.

Unfortunately, your addiction isn't your friend, and it certainly isn't something you can reason with. You might have the best excuse in the world, and nobody, including yourself, would blame you if you smoked. But you will still be smoking. You will have whatever problem it was that provided you with the good excuse – and you'll be back smoking, too.

Over the years, I have seen hundreds of people stop smoking: some stay stopped and some don't. Those who go back often have a good excuse, but those who don't have always got one or two as well. They usually say, 'Well, smoking wouldn't have helped me.' And they are right.

One lady had her handbag stolen a few weeks after stopping: and she smoked. Another had a miscarriage soon after she stopped: but she didn't smoke. One man had a close friend die in an accident a couple of months after he stopped: he didn't smoke.

Smoking just a few seems such a wonderful compromise. The one thing that will help you, *especially at difficult times*, is to remember what the stakes really are. You either choose to smoke all the cigarettes you would end up smoking year after year, or you choose, just for now, to smoke none of them.

After you've stopped smoking, your choice to light a cigarette is your choice to return to a life of smoking. After you stop, examine that option carefully and remember that it's still an option you have and always will have. You can go back to being a smoker, any time. All you need to do is light up one cigarette.

IN OTHER WORDS: GILLIAN

I smoked my first cigarette when I was 17. It made me feel dreadfully ill and I recall with dismay how hard I had to work at becoming an addictive smoker – and all in aid of being 'one of the group'. I persisted, and within six months I was on 20 a day.

Nineteen years and about 140,000 cigarettes later, I decided to quit, and I didn't smoke again for over two years. Cigarettes belonged to the past. I felt wonderfully well and in charge of my life. Then, at a party, someone offered me a Gauloise and I decided to have just one madly continental puff. Within six weeks I was back to 20 a day.

Twenty years and around 220,000 cigarettes later, I had a bad bout of bronchitis and a premonition of dying like this within a year. Instead, I did Full Stop.

If only I had known, 20 years earlier, the few simple techniques that are the key to the Full Stop method, I would never have risked that one puff.

CHAPTER 7

Why Smoking Seems to Help

I wonder if we could contrive . . . some magnificent myth that would in itself carry conviction to our whole community.

PLATO, *THE REPUBLIC*

At any time after you have stopped smoking, if you then choose to smoke, you choose to become a smoker again. Only when you take this fact into consideration do you gain the conviction it takes not to smoke that first one. But even though you know that smoking one means you smoke them all, there are other deceptions the addiction creates that can make it difficult not to take that first puff. These deceptions are the beliefs about smoking being helpful in various ways. We looked at this briefly in Chapter 2.

For example, you may imagine that nicotine contributes to your ability to do certain things, such as concentrate, make decisions or be creative; in other words, it helps you think. Or you may believe it helps you to cope with emotions that you otherwise would not be able to handle. In other words, smoking keeps you from hitting your kids or swearing at your boss.

Some people see cigarettes as their friends, perhaps the only consistent element in what seems to be an unreliable world. Others think that smoking gives them confidence or makes them socially more assured.

This is your psychological dependency. You believe that you are dependent on cigarettes, or nicotine, in order to live your life the way you do.

Stopping smoking is the process of breaking free from this dependency, and this means challenging the belief system you have developed which says that you need to smoke. After all, it's going to be tough to stay stopped if you cannot function in some crucial way without smoking.

The first point to grasp is this: just because you believe something doesn't make it true. It will be essential to acknowledge this in order to begin to see through these delusions and to overcome your dependency on cigarettes.

To prove this point, look at the following example. Many people, including the ship's captain, believed that the *Titanic* could not sink. Their conviction, however, didn't make it so: they held a false belief about it. Their belief was based on what seemed to them like sound evidence: the ship was said to have been constructed so as to be unsinkable.

In the same way, you probably have what seems to you to be good reasons for your beliefs, and you also jump to false conclusions. You are, in fact, attributing capabilities to nicotine that are far greater than its actual chemical effect. This is characteristic of any addiction.

It's usually easier to see how false these delusions are when you look from the outside into another person's dependency. The alcoholic believes that drink is making him more effective at work, but eventually he gets fired because of it. The woman who binges believes that by eating she can cheer herself up, but actually she is constantly miserable about how much rubbish she continues to eat.

The heroin addict gets a shot of self-esteem in the arm, but really the addiction leaves him feeling less than human.

In the same way, people who have never smoked look at you and puzzle about what smoking contributes to your life. You, on the other hand, are inside the dependency looking out, where it all seems very convincing. That's the whole problem: *you genuinely believe that you have to smoke in order to function well in your life.*

Like any other belief, if you tell yourself something over and over again for years and years, you will end up very convinced.

How the Delusions are Created

You develop these beliefs about smoking along with developing the addiction. They are part of the same process: the addictive desire is interwoven with your justification for satisfying it, reinforced over and over again. Like any other belief, if you tell yourself something over and over again for years and years, you will end up very convinced. And the more you feel deprived of smoking when you stop, the more convinced you will become.

Just as it took time for you to develop the delusion of dependency, so it takes time to work through it and break it down.

Let's take one example, to see how this happens. Look at the process of writing, whether it is letters, a report or a story. A smoker with this kind of dependency believes that smoking helps them to write, usually to the point where they are incapable of writing without it. So what is going on?

At some time, probably very early on in the addiction, you smoked a cigarette while writing. It only has to happen once to set up the conditioned reflex: after you have connected the activities of writing and smoking once, the association has been established. The next time you want to write something, you have a memory of smoking while writing. This triggers your desire to smoke. You respond to your desire by smoking, and this reinforces the connection once again.

Then, whenever you get to the end of a sentence and you aren't sure of what to write next, there's a desire to smoke. This gets satisfied and reinforced before the next sentence is written. The illusion that gets built up is that smoking helps you think of the next sentence. But in fact, all smoking does is temporarily satisfy your addictive desire.

Now, when you get around to stopping smoking, what happens is that the desire to smoke at the end of the sentence doesn't get satisfied. You may try to ignore it at first, perhaps by substituting mints or coffee, for example, to keep the desire at bay. But this doesn't work because mints and coffee don't satisfy a desire to smoke, and the desire becomes more and more of a problem. Concentration is completely lost as your focus is shifted from whatever you are writing to resisting the desire. So, finally, you return to smoking so that your concentration can be kept on the writing. And the belief that smoking is helping you to write is reinforced once again.

So what can you do about it? Wait until you never again need to write anything before you stop smoking? No, that won't work either, because you will have different delusions about how smoking helps, depending on what you are doing. Even if you are sitting around all day with nothing to do, you can become convinced, through exactly the same process, that smoking keeps you from feeling bored. You will always invent 'good' justifications for smoking; it's an automatic and inevitable part of being addicted.

What helps is to see that the justifications are false, whatever they are. And the only way to do that is to tackle them head on and question them as part of the process of stopping smoking. The techniques in Part Two will show you just how to achieve this. For the moment, it's important to see what the tricks are that your addiction can play.

All these delusions are created in much the same way. You meet a particular situation, and you smoke. From then on, you have a desire to smoke whenever you are in that situation again. You smoke the cigarette, which satisfies your desire, and you tell yourself a story about how the cigarette helped you with the situation. Tell yourself that story over many years and you have a powerful belief that you really do need to smoke in that kind of situation.

Delusions are also held in place because, when you first stop smoking, you experience withdrawal. For example, you will probably lose concentration during withdrawal, so smoking does improve your ability to concentrate in as much as it keeps you from experiencing a withdrawal symptom. It will help if you remember that withdrawal is a temporary phase: when it is over you will be able to think more clearly.

The Miracle Drug

If you study the delusions, you can begin to see how ridiculously varied and even contradictory they are. You may tell yourself that smoking wakes you up in the morning and also believe that it helps you get to sleep at night. You simultaneously believe that smoking helps you focus on something and that it distracts you from thinking about something unpleasant. You believe that smoking stops you from feeling hungry and also that it helps you to digest a meal you have just finished. Smoking seems to alleviate both boredom and stress. It's a mask to hide behind when you are unsure of yourself and a social tool to bring people together. It energises and relaxes you.

If you saw a product advertised claiming to do all these things, wouldn't you be just a little bit suspicious? The fact is you can believe that smoking does almost anything you want it to.

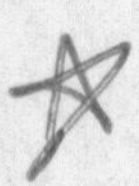

Or you can honestly admit that your dependency is an illusion and that the only thing smoking really achieves is to satisfy your addictive desire to smoke.

This is one of the truly empowering aspects of stopping smoking. You discover that you really are capable of doing all kinds of things you previously thought you owed to nicotine.

Magnificent Myths

Here are some of the most common delusions about smoking and some of the facts behind the myths.

'*Smoking helps me to control my emotions.*' You might believe that if you stop smoking an uncontrollable rage or desperate sadness will become unleashed. If this seemed to happen in past attempts to stop smoking, it was certainly the result of feeling deprived. You believed that you couldn't smoke any more, and you got angry and/or sad about that. But if you stay in touch with your choices – that you are always free to do whatever you want – all that negativity and hostility evaporates, without smoking.

Remember, though, that you have no doubt made an association with smoking whenever you got upset, angry, frustrated or depressed. So whenever you feel such strong emotions, you will have an intense desire to smoke. This is through the conditioned association, just as having a cup of coffee can trigger a desire to smoke. When you feel angry, you want to smoke. Lighting a cigarette satisfies that desire, and you think it has calmed you down.

In fact, far from calming you down, it excites your nervous system for a few seconds, making your heart race and your head swim. You use the buzz to distract you from whatever it is that is upsetting you, and tell yourself that smoking was essential and inevitable. But if you want to distract yourself from whatever it is you are angry about, you can do that in any number of ways without smoking. You don't need to smoke a cigarette in order to take a few moments to draw breath and gather your thoughts about the situation.

If you can acknowledge your free choice about whether or not you smoke, you will have put that crippling sense of deprivation behind you. Then you will find you are perfectly capable of dealing with your anger at least as effectively as you normally do, without smoking.

The same applies to depression. If you ever felt depressed as a smoker, then you know from your own experience that smoking doesn't cure depression. If anything, it makes it worse because you get depressed about your smoking. And the stress smoking puts on your body drains your energy, which further depresses your state of mind.

The solution lies in *expecting* the inevitable desire to smoke, which, admittedly, will be tough to deal with while you are angry or depressed. It's tough, but it's possible. If you can experience, just once, your anger or depression passing anyway, even without resorting to smoking, then you have begun to overcome your dependency, and accepting the desire will become increasingly easier.

What's important is to see that smoking doesn't really help; that you will have the desire, but that smoking just satisfies that desire. It doesn't satisfy you.

You will also feel your desire to smoke, by the way, when you are feeling wonderful. Seeing smoking as a way to celebrate something or prolong a feeling of happiness is an equally powerful delusion.

'*Smoking keeps my weight down.*' This is a very common justification for smoking, and we will take a whole chapter to discuss it. If weight is your main concern about stopping smoking, Chapter 13 will explain how to proceed.

'*I need the oral gratification.*' This phrase is particularly insidious because it sounds like a valid scientific description of some deep instinctive need. If you take it literally, the term simply means that you stick something in your mouth (oral) and you find it satisfying (gratification).

Whatever your addiction, you will always make a positive association with anything that's directly connected with getting your fix. If you were addicted to cocaine, you could become especially fond of any white powder, and of inhaling things up your nose. Heroin addicts actually get a thrill out of sticking needles in their veins.

However, most people using 'oral gratification' as an excuse are thinking of some far more essential need, apart from and deeper than the addiction or the superficial pleasure.

The theory behind this need for oral gratification, and what appears to give it authority, is the Freudian one that if a baby isn't weaned properly, it will forever after need a substitute. In other words, you can blame your mother for your smoking! But, as many mothers know, two babies can be nurtured in exactly the same way and one of them, as an adult, may end up smoking (or overeating, drinking, gambling, etc.) while the other one doesn't.

If you resent the circumstances of your life enough, you can justify doing almost anything.

A variation on this belief is that sucking on cigarettes compensates for a lack of love in your present life. It's so easy to blame your circumstances; if you resent the circumstances of your life enough, you can justify doing almost anything.

But if you look around, you will see that there are other people in the same, or worse, situation who don't smoke, and they are coping with the difficulties they face each day. The only difference between you and them is the addiction you have developed.

Cigarettes aren't your friends. They don't provide you with support; all they support is the addiction.

It may be you are not happy with things that are happening in your life, and it may be that some of those things are beyond your power to change at present. Your smoking, however, is something you always have the ability to control completely, no matter what anyone else says or does. In fact, it may be the one thing at this time that you can change – and the sense of achievement you get from stopping smoking could take you on to making changes in other circumstances.

Another belief you may hold is that you need to smoke for the same, unresolved reasons you gave yourself when you first started to smoke, many years ago. And you may think you need to discover what those reasons are and resolve them before you can successfully stop smoking.

But the important factor is *that* you chose to smoke, not why. All that is relevant to you now, in the process of stopping, are the reasons you give yourself now as to why you *continue* to smoke. These reasons may or may not be the same as the ones you gave when you started.

'*Smoking helps me to relax.*' You get home after a hard day's work and you sit down in your favourite, most comfortable chair with a drink and a cigarette. Smoking has helped you to relax and unwind after the day's hectic pace.

But has it? You have inhaled the lethal gas carbon monoxide in a concentration 600 times the safe level in industry. Along with that you have also inhaled 4,000 chemicals, many of them poisonous, including hydrogen cyanide, carbolic acid and arsenic trioxide.

Nicotine itself is a deadly poison and can be used as an insecticide. If you took the nicotine from one packet of cigarettes and injected it into your blood stream all at once, it would kill you. That's why, with every cigarette you smoke, your heart pounds away with 20 extra beats per minute. Part of the buzz effect you like so much is your body trying to cope with a poison that is constricting your blood vessels.

Smoking is a cause of stress, not a relief. The delusion that it helps you to relax comes about through the conditioned association. Wanting to relax or take a break triggers your desire to smoke. Smoking relieves this desire and gives you the impression that it helped you to relax.

Again, this delusion often gets reinforced during attempts to stop smoking. If you deny choice when you stop smoking you will feel deprived and end up more tense and stressed than when you were smoking. Then, of course, this stress is alleviated as soon as you light up a cigarette. You have demonstrated that you are free to smoke, so you no longer feel trapped. But you have also failed in your attempt to stop smoking – and reinforced your dependency as well.

The solution is to change the way you are thinking about choice during the process of stopping smoking. When you stay connected to the truth of free choice – whether or not you are actually smoking – you will feel much more relaxed. You will be able to notice your desire to smoke, but realise that it's your choice not to satisfy it. When you know that it's your free choice to do whatever you want to do, you can simply allow yourself to feel the desire rather than fight it.

'*Cigarettes give me energy.*' You will almost certainly have more energy after you've stopped smoking because every cell in your body will be healthier, with normal levels of oxygen in your blood. The nicotine buzz only seems to give you energy because it makes your heart race. Nicotine stimulates the release of adrenalin and cortisol, which are the stress hormones behind our 'fight-or-flight' response in emergencies. This produces a quick burst of energy, closely followed by tiredness. The energy lasts only seconds and then the effort expended and the chemicals ingested drag your energy level right down.

'*Smoking gives me something to do.*' Many smokers are concerned about what they will do to occupy themselves when they stop smoking. But this need not be a problem if you are willing to face, manage and accept the desire to smoke that lies behind it.

When you stop, there will be many gaps during your day where you would have smoked a cigarette. Your concern about these gaps is really your concern about feeling your desire to smoke. Your desire to smoke can be experienced in the form of wanting to pick up a cigarette and hold it, or wanting to fill an awkward or boring moment.

In fact, there is nothing particularly fascinating about smoking a cigarette. And your hands don't actually need to be occupied all the time. Just look at all the times during the day when you are not smoking: what do your hands do then? My guess is that you rarely think about what they are doing. When you've just stopped smoking, the only time you will think about them is when you are experiencing your desire to smoke.

The Placebo Effect

The truth is that all the help smoking seems to give you springs almost entirely from the placebo effect. A placebo is something that creates an effect, but the effect doesn't come from the placebo, it is created by your mind – as the following experiment demonstrates.

A group of 56 medical students were given either pink or blue pills containing nothing but a tiny bit of sugar and told that they had been given either a stimulant or a sedative. Of those who took blue pills, 72 per cent decided they must have been given sedatives because they felt drowsy. Pink pills had less of an effect, although 32 per cent of those who took them felt less tired, so they concluded that they had taken stimulants. *Only three students reported that the pills had no effect at all.* One third of the students reported side effects ranging from headaches, dizziness and watery eyes to abdominal discomfort, tingling extremities and staggering gait.[1]

If these reactions are made spontaneously to an inert substance, how much more likely it is that you will attribute extra capabilities to a drug like nicotine, which does have a chemical effect.

An interesting but probably unanswerable question is: where does the chemical effect stop and the placebo effect begin?

Certainly smoking immediately produces a faster heart rate, higher blood pressure and more adrenalin. A variety of other effects – ability to concentrate and memorise, for example – have frequently been examined, but so far no clear scientific evidence has appeared to support the belief that nicotine is a genuine aid to human life in any way.

Whatever it is that nicotine really contributes – other than satisfying an addiction to nicotine – is obviously fairly insignificant.

On the other hand, of course, smoking is frequently a nuisance and can hinder just as often as it seems to help. It takes up time and energy, and is something you continually need to think about and cater for. As a smoker, you are obliged to continue smoking at regular intervals in order to keep yourself from going into withdrawal. Far from being a crutch to assist you, it's really more like a ball and chain.

IN OTHER WORDS: IMOGEN

I had smoked for 10 years and given up many times, always returning after a few months when miserable, under stress or in a crisis. I hated and despised myself for smoking and felt my continual return to it meant that I was weak and despicable.

What I liked about Full Stop was that it carefully focused on smoking and the tricks we play with ourselves to stay addicted. Clearly separating out these smoking processes from all the other stress and distress in my life was a revelation and a relief.

Now, when I feel the urge to smoke, I don't say 'No, I mustn't have a cigarette.' I simply apply the technique. I am now acutely aware that all smoking a cigarette does is satisfy a desire to smoke; it doesn't actually help me feel better or solve a crisis.

The feelings of achievement, control, choice and empowerment are a continual source of pleasure to me. Many people have little sense of their own power, their ability to make choices and to act on them. An awareness of the fact of choosing to smoke or not can begin to release people from their self-imposed prisons and encourage them to take a more assertive, proactive and positive approach to life.

CHAPTER 8

The Motivation to Stop

For thy sake, tobacco, I would do anything but die.

CHARLES LAMB, *A FAREWELL TO TOBACCO*

A fundamental goal all of us, as living things, have in common is the goal of staying alive and in good health. Most of the primary functions of our minds and our bodies are, in fact, orientated towards helping us to survive and to live full lives.

Like most goals it is not reached in a single bound. An aeroplane doesn't fly in a straight line. It actually flies in a series of narrow zigzags. The plane veers off course, and is continually being corrected back on course again. Where the goal of our personal health is concerned, an addiction interferes with and distorts our natural process of course correction.

As a smoker, you will have already received lots of signals indicating that you are off course: a cough, a sore throat, loss of energy. These signals call softly at first, and unless you make the necessary course correction, they get louder and louder: chronic bronchitis, chest pains, high blood pressure . . .

The more you ignore the signals, the more off course you become. When you wake up with a smoker's hangover and 'cure' it by lighting a cigarette; when you notice your toes are numb from bad circulation and you go on smoking anyway; when you promise yourself you'll stop smoking next New Year's Eve, but you don't: all these result in a stronger and stronger commitment to that altered course.

Let's say that a plane leaves London for New York, and instead of heading south-west, it flies toward the south. The longer it takes for the correction to be made, the further away from its destination it gets. If this plane was a typical smoker, it would reason that it would be much better to get to Sydney, Australia, before making any changes!

This is what you are doing when you put off stopping smoking. Slowly but surely you reinforce your addictive behaviour by your procrastination. And the fundamental goal of your own health, vitality and self-esteem is bypassed and ignored.

Not Sure?

Usually, smokers rationalise by saying that they are not motivated to stop, or not motivated enough. *But what will it take for you to become motivated?*

Perhaps you are waiting for the addiction to go away, for the day when you wake up and don't feel the desire to smoke any more. But, as explained in Chapter 2, the desire to smoke doesn't go away. In fact, it gets more reinforced the longer you go on smoking. Some smokers find that smoking becomes less and less enjoyable, and even get to the point when they don't enjoy it at all, yet this still doesn't cancel out their addictive desire.

Perhaps you are waiting for some event to occur that will provide your motivation. Or until you have sorted the rest of your life out, whatever that may mean to you. But the only time you will be finished with that is when your life is over. Even more dangerous is to wait for your health to deteriorate to the point where you decide that you 'have to' stop. As we saw in Chapter 4, this kind of motivation is threatening, and because of the additional pressure it can actually make it more difficult for you to succeed.

It is often said that before anyone can successfully stop smoking, they must be completely convinced that they want to stop. That is a myth that keeps people smoking for decades. The idea of waiting for strong motivation to stop is a delusion fostered by your addictive thinking.

What is true is that most smokers deny the real seriousness of their situation, and inevitably approach stopping smoking with a lot of ambivalence. That's where much of the characteristic difficulty about stopping comes from. You are not completely sure that you want to stop, and you are not completely sure that you will be able to stay stopped. These two uncertainties often mix themselves up in your mind. You fear that you will never stay stopped, so you try to accept your life of smoking by telling yourself (and anyone who asks) that you don't really want to stop – *at least not now.*

Your motivation can also be compromised by fears about your dependency on cigarettes. If you fear that you will not be able to think clearly without smoking, then it will be hard to consider stopping at the risk, say, of losing your job. If you think that stopping smoking will make you put on a lot of weight, continuing to smoke may seem to be the preferable option. If you feel deprived when you stop, your self-pity and resentment will mask any benefits you may gain.

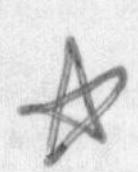

The truth is, you are attempting to do something that is vitally important to you, and quite challenging, with no way of knowing whether or not you will succeed.

The chances are that it's only when you begin to overcome these concerns that you will be able to appreciate that not smoking is a better way of life. But you can only overcome your fears by stopping smoking and handling the issues in the process.

So, when it comes to stopping smoking, don't make the mistake of waiting until you feel like doing it. *You may be waiting for a very long time.*

Even if you felt enthusiastic about stopping smoking at first, it's possible you won't allow yourself to feel it fully: partly because you are unsure how long it will last, and partly because being too enthusiastic might make you feel obliged to stay stopped. At the same time, somewhere deep inside, you certainly can be quietly delighted that you are, at least for now, not smoking.

Or you may be one of the few smokers who find it almost impossible to feel motivated to stop in any way. Obviously, you need to have *some* interest in stopping smoking, but be reassured – you don't need to feel like a cheerleader in order to succeed. If you handle the process of stopping correctly, your motivation to stay stopped will develop in time, quite possibly after periods of serious doubt and much debating with yourself.

A Gift to Yourself

If the main reason you are trying to stop smoking is because someone else is telling you or asking you to, you are holding them responsible for what you are doing. What you are saying, in effect, is: I don't care about my own well-being, but I'll do whatever you want me to do. This inevitably leads to feelings of deprivation. You are not making your own choices, so you experience stopping as an act of self-sacrifice, with consequent irritability and loss of any good motivation you might otherwise have had.

Stopping smoking could be the first truly 'selfish' thing you have ever done in your life.

It's very likely that you have, in fact, been asked to stop smoking by someone else, but that doesn't mean that this has to be your motivation now. What will work best for you is to put those people who want you to stop aside, in your mind, and focus on reasons that are for you and you alone.

This applies whether it's your parents, children, partner, friend, employer, doctor or just society in general who want you to stop.

This is one reason why I advised at the beginning of the book not to tell anyone that you're planning to stop, and to keep it quiet for as long as you can.

I suggest you make stopping smoking primarily a selfish thing you are doing for your own benefit. By 'selfish', I don't mean it will take anything away from anyone else. What I mean is that it's something you are doing to please yourself.

This can be a challenge, especially for the generation of older women who may have been brought up with the idea that they must always put others first. You might spend all your time looking after others, and think that the one thing in your day that you do for yourself is to smoke. It will be essential for you to see stopping smoking as your own personal choice to gain your own personal benefits, so that you don't end up feeling martyred. Stopping smoking could be the first truly 'selfish' thing you have ever done in your life.

A massive problem in stopping for others is that your ability to stay stopped becomes dependent on your relationship with those people. If at any time they do something that upsets or disappoints you, your motivation to stay stopped disappears. If you are stopping mainly because your workplace is now a no-smoking zone, you could be more likely to smoke when you're not at work. If you stop smoking so your children won't be passive smokers, you could be more likely to smoke when they're not around. If you stop smoking at your boyfriend's request, then you might stay stopped only up until the time you have an argument with him.

Another problem with stopping for someone else is that, even though they may be people that you love dearly, you can build a resentment towards them because you react emotionally as if they had taken away your cigarettes and forbidden you to smoke.

On the other hand, when you stop primarily because you have freely decided to make this change, you are taking responsibility for yourself, your own health and your own actions. You don't react as if someone has forced you into it. And – provided you remember you can always change your decision and return to smoking – you don't end up feeling deprived.

It is only when you stop smoking primarily for selfish motives, because it will result in an improved way of life for you, that you can get motivated and stay motivated. Staying stopped is now aligned with your own profound inner instincts for survival.

'I Might Get Run Over by a Bus'

Think for a moment about why you are prepared to stop smoking for someone else, but not for yourself. Why is it that they want you to stop, when you apparently don't? How can it be that you are content to go on smoking, but can't bear the thought of your children starting? And how can you possibly wish that someone else that you love would stop, while continuing to smoke yourself?

This is all possible because of an important aspect of the addiction: your well-practised ability to justify your own smoking. All the time you have been smoking, you have been bombarded by information about the dangers of what you are doing to yourself.

Most smokers defend themselves, both to themselves and to others, by creating a kind of mental buffer. It helps you to live with your addiction in the face of overwhelming evidence that it is one of the most self-destructive things you could be doing. You rationalise, hold beliefs that sound logical but are, in fact, completely flawed, and simply deny the more obvious truths.

The rationalisations and denial will be familiar to you, and the realities they cover up will be essential for you to face up to as part of the process of stopping. Here are some of the most common. As you read them, remember that the key to seeing through any of these lies is to remind yourself that you can always be a smoker, if that is what you choose to do with your life.

'*The damage is already done.*' This may well be true in very advanced stages of serious diseases, such as lung cancer or atherosclerosis. But your risk of getting smoking-related diseases like cancer or heart disease declines steadily after you have stopped. And if you already have emphysema, then when you stop smoking, it won't get any worse and whatever breathing capacity you have, you'll keep.

When people justify their smoking this way, what they may really be saying is that they have given up on themselves. This, of course, is a profound decision. And it is one you can reverse.

'*We're all going to die sooner or later.*' For smokers, it's sooner. According to a report based on information from every life insurance company in Britain, 'On average, a 45-year-old smoker is more than twice as likely to die before reaching 60 as a non-smoker of the same age.'[1]

If you are fairly young, it's possible that old age doesn't look particularly attractive to you, so you're not sure why you would want to prolong it. But as a smoker, you don't eliminate old age, you simply make it happen sooner. Smoking ages you more than anything else does, in both your external appearance and your internal health. As just one example, dermatologists have found wrinkles on the faces of 20-year-old smokers![2]

As a smoker, you don't eliminate old age, you simply make it happen sooner.

Yes, you might get run over by a bus tomorrow; nobody knows how long they will live. One thing you can be completely sure of, though, is that the quality of your health is already impaired, right now, by your smoking. The longer you smoke, the more serious that impairment will become.

'*I must have one little vice.*' Many people are able to stop drinking or can diet successfully, but think of cigarettes as their last straw to clutch on to. But you don't need to have any addictions at all: they serve no real purpose.

This 'it's my last straw' kind of rationalisation often comes from people who are doing a lot for others and spend too little time looking after themselves. If you can see that smoking isn't really a way of looking after yourself, perhaps, after you have stopped, you will want to find other ways of providing real support and rewards for what you do.

'*Smoking doesn't affect me, and I would stop immediately if it ever did.*' Smoking is affecting you now and it's only a matter of time before you will be made aware of it. For some people, the very first symptom they ever notice is a heart attack. But smoking was affecting them long before that happened.

Another form of denial is pretending that a symptom like shortness of breath is caused by something else, such as asthma or allergies. One way to challenge that pretence is to stop smoking for a while, and see what difference it makes.

As one doctor put it, many years ago: 'Addicts are usually unaware of their disturbance of judgement; thus many smokers will allege in all seriousness that their cough is due to damp, draughts, dust, fumes, infection, chill, "catarrh" or gas in the last war. They will take all manner of useless medications while rejecting and even resenting the suggestion that smoking might be responsible.'[3]

According to the US Surgeon General's report of 1990: 'It is safe to say that smoking represents the most extensively documented cause of disease ever investigated in the history of biomedical research.'

'*I don't really smoke.*' This is an excellent example of denial. A 30-a-day smoker who was terrified of getting cancer admitted to me that she was able to deny to herself the fact that she smoked. Fortunately, it has now really become true for her. This gives you some idea of the power of the mind to deceive when it comes to justifying addiction.

Many smokers lie to themselves – and others – about how much they smoke, and few want to keep track of how many years it has been since they started.

What It's Like to be an Ex-smoker

This list will help you to identify some of the specific ways in which the quality of your life improves after stopping.

Health statistics are a good source of information about the dangers of smoking, but your own experience will be far more relevant to you. After stopping, it's crucial to remember what it was like to be a smoker, and exactly what it cost you, in all kinds of ways.

It will be helpful for you to make a detailed list, so you can refer to it if you forget. Keep it somewhere safe – in this book or in a diary – because you will want to read it through much later on when you could be taking things a bit for granted.

Some frequently reported personal benefits are:

- More energy
- Improved sense of taste and smell
- Improved breathing
- Improved hearing
- Improved voice
- Clearer, less irritated eyes
- Cleaner, healthier teeth and gums
- Fresher breath
- Clearer thinking
- Feeling more relaxed
- Less sleep needed
- Wake up feeling better
- Improved blood circulation: warmer fingers and toes

- Improved blood pressure
- Fewer headaches
- No sore throat
- No wheezing or smoker's cough
- No more pains in chest or legs
- Better chance of a longer and more active life
- Much lower risk of emphysema
- Much lower risk of circulatory problems
- Diminished risk of many cancers, especially lung, larynx and oral cavity
- Lower risk of stroke
- Later onset of osteoporosis (brittling of the bones)
- Less risk of gastric and duodenal ulcers
- Less heartburn and acid indigestion
- Lower risk of pneumonia and bronchitis
- Reduced risk during a general anaesthetic
- Lower risk from other drugs and medications, such as contraceptive pills
- Fewer allergy and sinus problems
- Fewer and shorter colds
- Improvement in existing problems such as asthma, diabetes and emphysema
- Later onset and fewer problems during the menopause
- Lower risk of male impotence
- More satisfying experience of sex
- Improved sports performance
- More active and productive
- More money
- Better job opportunities
- Better insurance rates
- Freedom from restrictions on smoking
- No more standing outside in the cold to smoke

- Cleaner home and car
- No burnt clothes or furniture
- No more smelly ashtrays
- Less risk of starting a fire
- Safer driving
- Great sense of accomplishment
- No more fears about the consequences of smoking
- No more guilt about smoking
- No longer obsessed with the need to stop smoking
- Freedom from dependency
- Increased self-confidence and self-respect
- No longer smelling like a smoker
- No nicotine stains on fingers
- Looking younger
- Improved complexion
- Fewer wrinkles
- Improved scar healing
- Feeling in control
- Desire and confidence to make other positive changes
- More positive view of life

This is not a complete list! There is, for instance, a large number of serious physical conditions that smoking either creates or makes worse. There is no part of your body that smoking does not affect because it keeps high levels of poisonous chemicals in your blood stream, and blood supplies every cell in your body. This happens with every cigarette you smoke, from the very first. It's just a matter of time before the symptoms get dramatic, but smoking affects you long before that.

The difference in the healing of scars is interesting because it is so easily measured. A study was made of a group of women undergoing the same minor routine operation. The group of 120 included 69 smokers. After healing, the smokers' scars were almost three times as wide as those of the non-smokers.[4]

Can You Expect Immediate Results?

There is, of course, no way to guarantee that you will get all the benefits you hope for straight away. Sometimes, for example, people anticipate having more energy when they stop, and are disappointed to find it doesn't seem to increase much at all. This actually depends on your level of fitness. Smokers who engage in sport or regular exercise almost always find their endurance improves after they stop smoking. They can easily measure it in terms of laps swum or squash games played and won. Often, those people who say they don't feel any fitter are not at all fit to begin with. Stopping doesn't make you fit; what it does is to vastly improve your ability to increase your level of fitness.

The speed of improvements in health will also depend on how much you've smoked, and for how long. The more damage done, the longer it can take for your body to recover. Different bodies react in different ways: some people feel very much better from the day they stop, and others take a long time, perhaps six months, before they can notice any improvement in their health.

But of all the benefits of stopping, the most commonly felt that my clients have told me about is derived from feeling free from dependency, and this happens almost at once. They experience an enormous thrill from being in control of their addiction for the first time in years.

Many people gain a few unexpected benefits from stopping. When I stopped smoking, I was very surprised by how much more alive I felt in the mornings and that I no longer felt sleepy in the afternoons. One recent client found that her chronic lower back pain disappeared within a week of stopping. Another client was amazed to find she didn't need to wear glasses any longer. Another, after 35 years of smoking, was surprised by the smell of a pencil.

It is important, however, especially in the first few weeks of stopping, to look honestly at the difference not smoking is making to you and to remember what smoking was really like. In particular, don't underestimate the peace of mind you will have when you are free from the habitual fear and guilt you have lived with as a smoker.

Finally, if you really don't see any improvement in your life at all, remember you can always go back to being a smoker. I have always found that whenever anyone truthfully considers the options open to them, they soon get in touch with their real motivation to stay stopped. You could decide that you really do want to be a smoker, but just remember the whole package that goes with this deal. It's up to you!

In Part Two, we will describe in detail how to work with the benefits that apply personally to you, to support you to stop, and stay stopped for good.

IN OTHER WORDS: JANE

I remember my first cigarette well. I was 15, on holiday in Scotland, and lit up a St Moritz menthol complete with gold band to impress Stuart from Glasgow – a glamorous creature of 18 or so. Stuart was unmoved, but I had taken my first step towards a 60-a-day romance with smoking that was to last for 20 years.

In all that time I never even tried to give up smoking. I loved it. It gave me 'confidence'. It was 'sophisticated'. Bedridden with bronchitis, I still managed 30 a day and it was an unusual Saturday night that did not involve a 4 a.m. trek to some distant all-night store to replenish supplies.

I went to Full Stop as a journalist, just as an observer, with no intention of giving up and a sceptical view of the claims made for the course. One week later I was an ex-smoker, still a doubtful one, but I had passed my first 24 hours in a decade without a cigarette. And as one smoke-free day led to another, I had to concede that perhaps I really had stopped.

Three years later I still haven't smoked, and though I still experience the occasional desire to do so, I am astonished by the relative painlessness of the process. That Full Stop truly works is borne out for me by the fact that I had not passionately wanted to stop – and had never for one moment thought I could anyway. Full Stop is a remarkable technique that took me by surprise.

Part Two
A Skill You Can Learn

CHAPTER 9

Changing Your Mind

Reason does not work automatically: thinking is not a mechanical process . . . The function of your stomach, lungs or heart is automatic; the function of your mind is not. In any hour and issue of your life, you are free to think or to evade that effort.

AYN RAND, *ATLAS SHRUGGED*

Now that you understand more about the nature of your addiction, Part Two will focus on the practical aspects of how to train your mind to manage your experience of wanting to smoke. These techniques are aids to changing your thinking. They won't do the work for you: they are tools for you to use.

It's helpful to understand how the technique works while you are still smoking, so it's a good idea to read through these chapters before you stop. But you can only use it properly after you have stopped because it's not possible to develop the skill of managing your desire to smoke while you are still satisfying it with cigarettes.

As with any other skill, like swimming for example, a certain amount can be explained first, and then there comes a point when you can learn no more until you face your fears and get into the water.

The first step is to recognise that after you stop smoking, you will experience your desire to smoke. These are your only options: you either go on smoking, or you learn how to cope with the unsatisfied desire to smoke.

The desire will fade in time, becoming less and less frequent, and much less intense. But it's not the infrequency of your desire to smoke that will help you to stay stopped. What makes the difference in the long term is how you cope with it when it's there. *The process of stopping smoking is the process of learning how to manage your desire to smoke.*

When you manage your desire to smoke, you can live alongside it. You notice that it's there from time to time but it doesn't make you smoke. In order to do that, your mind needs to be consciously retrained by you.

Outlined here is everything you need to know in order to manage your desire for a cigarette whenever it occurs. While you are smoking, your desire has been connected, thousands of times over, with smoking a cigarette. Now, a new connection is being established: your desire to smoke becomes your cue to think.

The Outline

- 'I have a desire to smoke.'

  As soon as you are aware of a desire to smoke, begin by paying attention to it, instead of trying to distract yourself. Facing your desire doesn't mean you want to go back to being a smoker. It simply enables you to identify what is happening and gain some time for yourself to think.
- 'I have the freedom to smoke!'

  You could make a choice to return to smoking. If you

don't deliberately remind yourself of this, it's likely you will assume you can't smoke and so create difficult symptoms of deprivation.

- 'One puff, and I'll be smoking.'

  Word by word, you spell out the simple truth: you are always just a puff away from connecting with the full force of your addiction again, as we saw in Chapter 6.

- Either: 'I choose to return to smoking.' Or: 'For now I choose to accept this desire rather than return to smoking.'

  Now there's a choice for you to make. Try saying to yourself: 'I choose to return to smoking,' and see if it's what you really want to do. Alternatively, choose to accept the feeling of unsatisfied desire.

  Choosing for now is a reminder that you are not making one choice to last for ever. You accept the desire just as it is right now, even if it feels very uncomfortable. The more times you can let yourself feel your unsatisfied desire to smoke, the easier it will become to do this.

  The more you accept the thoughts and feelings of desire, completely and unconditionally, the better. You will be more likely to succeed in the long term and you will have less difficulty in doing so. See Chapter 11 for more on this.

- 'I'm choosing this in order to gain these benefits . . .'

  Finally, complete the process by reminding yourself of the benefits to you in stopping smoking. Which is the most significant to you might change from day to day. Chapter 8 will help you to identify what these benefits might be for you.

Here is the whole process outlined in one sequence:

The Outline

How to Make a Choice

I have a desire to smoke
I have the freedom to smoke
One puff and I'll be smoking
Either:
I choose to return to smoking
Or:
For now, I choose to accept this desire
So I can enjoy these benefits from not smoking . . .

Making it Real for Yourself

It's important to consider each of the statements in The Outline. It's common to have doubts about them at first, because this is part of the process, but the idea is to spend some time thinking about them. Just saying the words parrot-fashion, without any conviction at all, isn't going to help you.

In order to help you make The Outline authentic, I suggest, as I suggest to all my clients, that you keep cigarettes with you during the first couple of weeks after you stop smoking. Don't hide away from the reality of your desire and freedom of choice. Instead, have packets of your favourite brand around you, with matches, lighters and ashtrays, just as they usually are, at work, at home and when you are socialising. Have an open pack of your cigarettes right in front of you, whenever you feel the desire to smoke; you could even hold it in your hands.

You might find it helpful to talk to the packet, holding a dialogue with the addiction. It's as if the addiction is talking to you, and in order to stay stopped you learn how to talk back to it.

The more uncomfortable you feel about carrying cigarettes, the more resistant you are to making the necessary changes in your thinking. When you have real cigarettes in front of you, you will face your real desire to smoke, you will learn how to manage it, and you will be able to reaffirm your freedom of choice in a real and lasting way.

It's as if the addiction is talking to you, and in order to stay stopped you learn how to talk back to it.

Carrying cigarettes is the part of the technique that some clients object to most strongly when they first hear about it, but later say it is the part they appreciate the most. It makes an enormous difference, because it immediately breaks down the panic, anxiety and misery of thinking you have trapped yourself in a state of deprivation. It's the best and fastest way to become genuinely confident that you can be in control of your addiction, and stay in control.

The main objection to carrying cigarettes, of course, is that in a weak moment you will smoke one. But if you stop smoking with cigarettes at hand, you can overcome your fear that your desire to smoke will overpower you and make you do something you didn't really want to do. *Understand that it's not your desire to smoke that makes you smoke. It's the inevitable consequence of your unwillingness to manage and accept the feeling of the desire.*

If your ability to stay stopped depends on not having cigarettes within reach, then you may not stay stopped for long. You are living in a world where there are cigarettes, people are going to be smoking them, even offering them to you, and there is no doubt that you will have some desire to smoke them sooner or later.

This is from a study of relapsed smokers: 'Other smokers serve not only as cues for smoking but as sources of cigarettes. In half of all relapsed episodes, another smoker provides the cigarettes that are smoked . . . in most cases the ex-smoker specifically asks for a cigarette.'[1]

Unconscious Smoking

Using The Outline is the way to manage your desire to smoke so that you gain conscious, deliberate control over your smoking, without the danger of starting again unintentionally.

As a smoker, it's very likely you smoke in an unconscious way quite often, unaware that you have lit a cigarette because you had your mind on something else. It's common and entirely understandable to fear that this might happen after you have stopped.

If you were to try and stop by evading and avoiding your desire, it would be much easier to suddenly and unconsciously light a cigarette, and you may even have done that in past attempts to quit. You stopped smoking, you were doing okay, you began to feel that maybe you'd succeeded this time, and then suddenly (oh, no!) you were smoking and had failed again.

This is why it's crucial to train yourself to notice and acknowledge your desire. Your desire to smoke can be ignored, but it lives on in your subconscious, and as soon as it begins to surface it immediately drives you to smoke automatically. There is no possible way for you to be in control of what you are doing because it's all happening below your conscious awareness.

The more time you put into using this technique, consciously repeating The Outline to yourself, the less likely it is that you will smoke without thinking about what you're doing.

Some people are especially good at repressing, even though they appreciate it's not helpful. They will find stopping smoking quite easy but will be very likely to return to smoking in this thoughtless way, regretting it afterwards but lighting that first cigarette blindly. If you have a tendency to repress, Chapter 11 explains how to induce desire, which will be an essential technique for you to gain lasting control.

When you stop smoking by acknowledging and accepting your desire to smoke, your conscious mind soon gets accustomed to noticing and coping with it.

Even so, you may still fear you'll smoke unconsciously after you've stopped, totally unaware of what you're doing. If this is a big concern for you, here are some things you can do in preparation:

- Make sure you can't get to a cigarette without first noticing what you're about to do. You can still have cigarettes available in the house, at your office, in your car. You simply create some kind of barrier so that you don't light one up *unconsciously.*
- You could tape the pack closed, put rubber bands or string around it, or keep it in a small bag or box. Be creative and figure out something that's right for you.

- If anyone else smokes in your household or office, and you are likely to smoke theirs, ask them to keep their pack of cigarettes to themselves and not leave them lying around. (If you are keeping quiet about stopping smoking, you could perhaps tell them that you want to know how many you are smoking, and so only want to take cigarettes from your own packet.)

Don't be surprised if you sometimes forget that you've stopped smoking and go to light a cigarette. At some point, however, you'll realise that you have stopped. Then you notice your desire to smoke and manage that desire by thinking through The Outline. At that point you make a conscious decision either to return to smoking or to accept your feeling of desire for that moment.

When you are a smoker, smoking another cigarette in an endless line of thousands is a relatively insignificant thing for you to be doing. After you have stopped smoking, however, lighting a cigarette becomes highly significant.

In Your Dreams

An entirely different kind of unconscious smoking is the smoking you might be doing in your dreams. It's quite common, after you have stopped, to dream you are smoking and wake up unsure whether it really did happen. This can be upsetting at first, but a great relief when you realise it was only a dream.

Dreaming about smoking doesn't mean you are not handling things effectively in your conscious, waking life, and it certainly doesn't indicate that you are going to relapse. All it means is that smoking is very much on your mind. Your dreams are just another way of working through the process of stopping.

The Line of Most Resistance

When it comes to stopping smoking, you can expect resistance all the way: it's part of the process. Before you stop, you might try to think of every excuse under the sun to go on smoking just a little bit longer. When you do stop, and you begin to work on staying stopped, there are a few more tricks your addicted mind can come up with to resist making any real changes.

You might try to think of every excuse under the sun to go on smoking just a little bit longer.

Forgetting The Outline. It's quite possible that you will completely forget a line or two of The Outline. The addicted part of your mind resists acknowledging the truth by simply blanking it out! This is one reason why it's important to say The Outline over and over again, not just to understand the theory behind it.

It's a good idea to write The Outline down and keep it with you at all times during the first few days of not smoking. The back of a business card works well, and you could keep it with your cigarettes. Then, if you have forgotten what to say to yourself, you can always read it.

Eventually you will want to memorise it so you can think it through at any time. Your desire to smoke will come and go, and you will always know how to cope with it when it's there.

Changing The Outline. A more subtle piece of resistance is to change the wording of The Outline by saying: 'I choose not to smoke.' When you make choices 'not to smoke', you say nothing about what it is that you are doing. You could, for example, manage to not smoke for a while by resenting or even repressing the desire to smoke. It is important to remind yourself that the way you stay stopped is to make choices 'to accept the desire'.

Believing you are too busy. Resistance also comes in the form of deciding you are 'too busy' to think about your desire to smoke. If you are a busy person, it will be important to make stopping smoking a priority for the first few weeks.

This means deliberately taking the time to manage your desire to smoke. It takes less than 30 seconds to go through the whole Outline, very carefully. You will find it is actually easier to keep taking the time to deal with your desire than to push it aside. You will be and feel much more in control if you make a clear choice to accept it each time.

If you keep using the technique, it will work: if you don't use it, you can find yourself in difficulty.

If you find you are having a desire to smoke during a conversation with somebody, on the phone for example, then first of all finish the conversation. Then, at the earliest opportunity, think through The Outline to yourself before you start anything else.

It's a mistake to tell other people what you are thinking and feeling when you have a desire to smoke: make it your own decision to accept your desire. It can be helpful to say The Outline out loud if you are alone, but my advice is to deal with your desire privately, especially at first while you are integrating the technique into your everyday life. When you discuss this with others you invite their comments, and that can be unhelpful.

How to Recognise the Desire

The desire to smoke can be just a thought, and it can also be a physical sensation. At first, the desire will be quite persistent but after a couple of days it should become obvious to you that it is triggered in your mind by events and circumstances, and not by any physical need.

Even though it is created in your mind, the desire is usually experienced as a physical sensation that leaves you feeling quite uncomfortable. You may well notice the physical sensation before fully realising what it is. When you first stop smoking, it can feel like a wave of discomfort all over your body. Later on, after you have stopped for a while, it can be similar to that sinking feeling you get when you realise, for instance, that you've locked your keys in the car.

Different people feel their desire to smoke in different ways, in different parts of their bodies. You might feel it in your chest area or throat, remembering the feeling of the smoke going into your lungs. You might feel the desire in your stomach and confuse it with hunger, or it may be more like wanting to put something into your mouth. Some people salivate more than usual when they want to smoke.

The form of your desire can change from day to day. In general, as time goes on, it will become less of a physically uncomfortable feeling and more like a thought. If you let yourself have these uncomfortable feelings and thoughts, then you will be able to stop smoking and stay stopped for good. If you don't, you won't: it's as simple as that.

It will be very much easier for you to accept when you remember that you are choosing to feel it, because, as far as you are concerned, it is better than the alternative of a life of smoking. This is just as important to remember months after you have stopped as it is during your first day of stopping.

IN OTHER WORDS: IRENE

I had previously tried to stop smoking by cutting down gradually over a period of time. I realise now that I was trying to get rid of the desire – and why I was so unsuccessful! I thought at first that these techniques would also help me get rid of the desire and that because I was still having these feelings I couldn't be using The Outline properly. I'm one of those people whose pain threshold is very low and I'll do anything to avoid it and protest loudly if I can't. Among other things, what The Outline requires is that you accept the pain! This idea had never occurred to me before. For me, it made all the difference when I acknowledged the desire instead of being frightened that I would immediately have a cigarette. In other words, I had a choice.

What helped the most was when I treated the desire – the voice nagging at me to have a cigarette – like a little child who needs attention. All the child needed was not to be ignored but to be given sympathy, love and attention.

CHAPTER 10

Starting Stopping

Think of me as one, even when four months had passed, still agitated, writhing, throbbing, palpitating, shattered; and much, perhaps, in the situation of him who has been racked . . .
THOMAS DE QUINCEY, *CONFESSIONS OF AN ENGLISH OPIUM EATER*

Withdrawal is your initial transition from being a smoker to being an ex-smoker. It is the most difficult part of stopping smoking, and the first question you probably have is: when will it end? You may have heard various estimates – from two days to four weeks – but there is no one answer that applies to everybody.

Symptoms coming from physical detoxification can become magnified and prolonged by your attitude.

First of all, it partly depends on how much you have smoked, and for how long. In general, if you have only smoked for five years you will experience less withdrawal than if you have smoked for 50. There are, however, individual variations.

How long withdrawal lasts also depends on how you are coping mentally with the process of stopping. Symptoms coming from physical detoxification can become magnified and prolonged by your attitude, so what would have been a very temporary difficulty becomes a persistent threat to your ability to stay stopped.

The most convincing proof of this comes from studies of smokers who experience the symptoms of withdrawal even though they have nicotine in their systems. And, making the same point in another way, there's a study of smokers whose withdrawal symptoms disappeared when they smoked, even though the cigarettes they were given were in fact nicotine-free.[1]

Some Common Symptoms

- Feeling light-headed, dizzy and disorientated. This is mostly due to the presence of a great deal more oxygen in your blood than you are used to, and it's actually a sign that your circulation is improving. The carbon monoxide in cigarette smoke inhibits your blood's ability to carry oxygen and the resulting increase in blood oxygen levels after you stop smoking is most noticeable in your brain. Occasionally this may affect your ability to think and concentrate clearly. This effect is variable from person to person, but for most people it starts to improve after the first day or two. By then your brain has readjusted to the new levels of oxygen, resulting in increased mental alertness.
- Excess hunger. For a great many smokers, their desire for a cigarette when they first stop smoking feels like an appetite for food. This is an important issue and we will look at it in detail in Chapter 13.
- Tingling sensations. If your circulation has been badly affected by your smoking, you may feel tingling sensations, especially down your arms and legs, for a day

or two after stopping. As nicotine constricts your blood vessels, your blood flows more freely when you stop smoking, and this change sometimes feels strange at first.

- Constipation. This can be a serious and persistent problem for some ex-smokers. Nicotine artificially stimulates the action of the bowels, as many smokers know, and some people have come to rely on smoking as the way to 'get them moving'. Over a long period of time, the bowels depend more and more on nicotine, so the ex-smoker can become constipated. By far the best remedy is a combination of water, exercise and the water-soluble fibre contained in vegetables and fruit.
- Losing sleep. It's fairly common for people to have interrupted sleep patterns when they have first stopped smoking. Be patient and this will correct itself. Understand that you have been using a stimulant drug and your body will take a bit of time to get back to its natural daily rhythms of energy and sleep at the appropriate times.
- Difficulty getting to sleep. Another physical effect of getting nicotine out of your system comes from the fact that caffeine has a stronger effect on you and stays in your body longer. If you feel tense after you stop smoking, try cutting down on your caffeine intake, and see if that makes a difference. If you have difficulty getting to sleep, try avoiding caffeinated drinks in the late afternoon and evening. Note that coffee, tea and many soft cola drinks all contain caffeine, and their 'decaffeinated' versions do as well. Many painkillers and premenstrual medications also contain high levels of caffeine.

- Increased sensitivity to alcohol. Alcohol can also have a stronger effect on you, so that you get tipsy faster on less. Some clients of mine report this effect to begin with, and a few tell me it seems to be a permanent change.
- Excess catarrh. Your nose can run because your sinuses are draining properly for the first time since you started smoking. Also, you may cough up nasty stuff from your lungs. Unpleasant as it seems, these are both signs of your improving health.
- Bad taste. Some people experience a nasty taste in their mouth when they first stop smoking. This same taste was there when you smoked: when you stop smoking, your taste buds come back to life and so you become aware of it.
- Sore throat. Your throat may feel sore when you first stop. Smoking makes your throat sore, but as it also numbs your whole sinus area, you only begin to feel it after you have stopped.

If these kinds of symptoms are very persistent, they may indicate a more significant problem and you should consult your doctor.

Your State of Mind makes All the Difference

By far the most problematic symptoms of withdrawal come from the ways in which you are thinking about smoking and not smoking. *It's not possible to have no attitude at all.* What attitude you take is what makes all the difference to your process, how traumatic it is and how successful you will be.

When you first stop smoking, assuming you are not avoiding and repressing, you can expect your desire to smoke to be fairly constant for about two days. For some people it's continuous and for others it comes and goes in waves. The second day is often more intense than the first.

During this time, you may also be quite disorientated, so you end up feeling rather peculiar, to say the least. After these two days (variable from person to person) you will see the desire begin to diminish.

The people I have worked with who just experience their desire, and nothing else, are willing to accept it as a temporary phase and don't see it as a problem. It doesn't have to feel like hell.

Extensive research on stress points to lack of choice as the principal cause.

Problems arise if, when they feel the desire for a smoke, people tell themselves they can no longer satisfy it. They deny choice, and they do that because they think that to acknowledge the freedom to smoke means they will smoke. The challenge is to fully acknowledge that the option of smoking exists – without actually doing it.

If you feel any of the following symptoms of deprivation after you stop smoking, then you have not yet changed the way you are thinking in this regard:

Desire to smoke doesn't diminish. Even a week after stopping, you still feel an intense and persistent desire, perhaps for hours on end, because the one thing you think you 'can't' have is the one thing you want the most.

Stress. Take a look at this list of symptoms: loss of temper, loss of sense of humour, loss of concentration, difficulty making decisions, 'cotton wool' head, tiredness not relieved by sleep, insomnia, indigestion, overeating, depression, headaches, heart palpitations, chest pains, heartburn, trembling, leg cramps, twitching in limbs.

I copied this list from a book, but it wasn't a book about smoking, it was a book about stress. It's not a complete list. Stress will show up in different ways in different people – depending on your Achilles heel.

The most important thing to understand about stress is that the symptoms are often psychosomatic: physical problems with causes created by a state of mind. Extensive research on stress points to lack of choice as the principal cause. If you have a desire and you tell yourself you can't smoke, you are guaranteed to create symptoms of stress, especially:

- Irritability: which may really be repressed rage.
- Anxiety: like a caged wild animal you become restless, anxious and can even reach a state of panic. Symptoms of panic attacks are: palpitations, difficulty in breathing, dizziness, hot and cold flushes, sweating and trembling.
- Tension: fighting the desire can create aches in neck, shoulders and stomach, nausea and difficulty relaxing.
- Depression: which could be seen as a form of repressed anger. Some of the symptoms are: loss of energy, apathy, early-morning waking, inability to concentrate or make decisions.

Getting Free, Staying Free

Freedom is a basic requirement of all living creatures. It is more important to you than almost anything else, certainly more important than stopping smoking. If, after you have stopped, you don't feel genuinely free to smoke, you will feel deprived until you get free.

If you are having difficulty grasping a real sense of choice, it will help you to discover what it is that makes you think you can't smoke. Some of the beliefs that give rise to feelings of deprivation are covered in Chapter 4, and you might identify with one or more of these. Or you may have your own, unique circumstance that leaves you feeling convinced that you don't have a real choice about this. If it is particularly difficult for you to overcome this issue, here is an exercise you can use to identify the thinking that supports your false belief and turn it around.

WRITTEN EXERCISE TO DEVELOP A GOOD SENSE OF FREE CHOICE

Please note: make sure you complete both *Step One and Step Two.*

Step One

If you are currently still smoking, write down:

'I have to stop smoking because . . .' and complete the sentence with as many different endings as you can think of. For example: '. . . if I don't, I'll die.' Or: '. . . otherwise I will hate myself.'

Leave one line blank in between each sentence ending.

If you have already stopped smoking and are feeling deprived, write down:

'I can't go back to smoking because . . .' and finish that sentence in as many different ways as you can. For example: '. . . if I do, I will have failed.' Or: '. . . if I do I'm afraid I'll never stop again.'

Leave one line blank in between each sentence ending. Be creative and find as many endings as possible, even those that seem outrageous or absurd.

Step Two

This is the crucial step, because it liberates you from your false belief. Go over your sentences, examine every line, and remind yourself that you are still free to smoke anyway. *The reasons you have listed are the consequences that you get, or might get, from choosing the option of smoking; they do not mean the option of smoking does not still exist. Write this in on the lines you have left blank. For example: ' If I don't stop, smoking might kill me, but I still could go on smoking.' Or: ' If I go back to smoking, I will have failed in my attempt to stop, but I'm still free to do that.'*

The very act of writing it down will be highly effective in reinforcing this new thinking. Repeat this exercise as often as you need.

Smoking is not an advisable choice, it's a disastrous option for you to take and quite possibly one that you desperately hope you don't take. But that never means it's not an option that is always available to you.

Whenever you pause to consider your options you access a particular area of your brain, a special part of your prefrontal cortex. This is why acknowledging free choice makes such a profound difference to the whole process of stopping smoking. It's good to consider your options any time at all, but especially helpful when you feel your desire to smoke. Consider what it would be like to return to smoking and remind yourself that this is up to you to choose how you want to live your life. Soon you'll begin to trust yourself to make choices that you really do want to live with.

Focus on choosing only for the present time. Consider that most of the resistance to getting in touch with your freedom to smoke is your fear that if you really can smoke, then you will! (Go back to Chapter 5 for clarification on making choices only in the present time.) This is especially helpful during the withdrawal phase. The more you make choices only for now, the less deprived you will feel, because then you are keeping your options wide open.

The simple key is to remember you are totally free to smoke – *and you don't have to do it to prove it!*

You Only Withdraw Once

Withdrawal is the essential first step to stopping smoking. For most smokers it is quite a challenge and it's helpful to have realistic expectations about it. If you think that it will be, or that it should be, effortless and easy, then you may very well be in for a nasty surprise. But if you prepare yourself for a challenge, and if you are prepared to deal with all the deceptions your addicted mind will produce, then you will emerge from the withdrawal phase successfully, and find staying stopped easier and easier to cope with.

Be encouraged by the fact that, if it is dealt with correctly, withdrawal is a temporary, one-off event. As soon as the changes have been made, both physically and mentally, they are over and done with and you will never need to go through anything like that again.

You Do Have A Choice

A

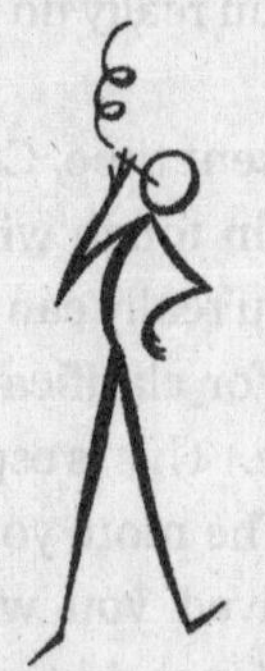

'I do have the freedom to smoke and I'm smoking.'
Many smokers think that when they stop smoking, that will be it – they will never smoke again. This once-and-for-all decision would make them feel deprived, as if they had lost their freedom to smoke (B), so they continue to smoke in order to feel free.

The more a smoker believes 'I have got to stop smoking', the more stopping will seem like deprivation and the more they look for excuses to continue.

B

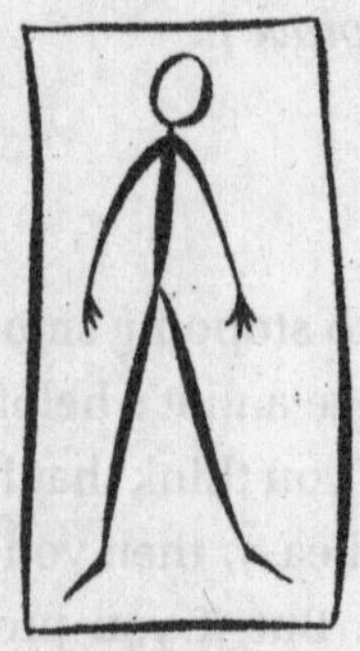

'I don't have the freedom to smoke.'
If, after you have stopped smoking, you deny that you could return to smoking, you will experience feelings of deprivation. This feels *as if* someone had locked you up and taken your cigarettes away (so you really wouldn't have a choice). You may feel resentful, angry, apathetic and/or martyred, but mostly you just want to get free.

The feelings of deprivation are very difficult to live with, so you either get free by smoking (A) or by changing your thinking (C). The exercise on page 131 will help you with this second option.

C

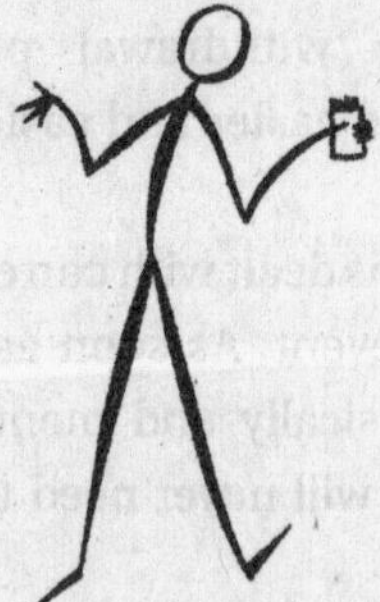

'I have the freedom to smoke, and I'm not smoking.'
It is possible to stop smoking and not feel deprived at all, even though you remember times when smoking was enjoyable and seemed helpful. Keep cigarettes with you so you can really believe you have the choice to smoke. Don't tell people that you have stopped smoking and if they ask, let them see that you have cigarettes and say something vague, like, 'I may have one later.' This keeps you in touch with your freedom to return to smoking, which means you won't feel deprived.

IN OTHER WORDS: BRIAN

I remember my first cigarette. I was in the woods of the local golf course with three or four other 15-year-olds. The first drag made me feel sick and giddy. But, like an idiot, I stuck with it and pretty soon I was indeed stuck with it – a 25-a-day habit that would, over the following 23 years, cost me thousands of pounds, make me smell revolting, and give me a wheeze that sounded like the massed pipes of the Royal Navy.

I'd tried giving up just once, on National No-Smoking Day. By 11 o'clock I was a wreck. By ten past I was smoking. So I trotted out the usual smokers' excuses: it's the pressure of my work . . . I don't really smoke that many . . . it's just something to do with my hands . . . I couldn't have a drink or a meal without a cigarette.

At first I was wary of the Full Stop programme. I figured that it was just a mind game, a trick. But reluctantly I started to focus on the choice that comes with every cigarette, eliminating the automatic flipping open of my pack of Rothmans. Did I really want to go on smoking? Wouldn't I prefer to give up coughing and wheezing? I started to deal with my habit one moment at a time. Logic entered into a subject that had always been dealt with on an emotive basis. I started to feel in control. The first few weeks were tough, but recognising that feeling uncomfortable was a critical and positive part of the quitting process made all the difference.

Now, some three and a half years later, the choice of whether to smoke or not arises far less frequently, and has become much easier to deal with. I don't feel smug – just pleased. I'm in control of my life and I'm not smoking – not at the moment.

CHAPTER 11

Taking Control

Living structures can only be if they become; they can exist only if they change. Change and growth are inherent qualities of the life process.

ERIC FROMM, *TO HAVE OR TO BE?*

As a smoker wanting to stop smoking, you are in a state of conflict. On one hand, you have an addictive desire to smoke. On the other, you want to stop satisfying it by smoking. Stopping smoking and staying stopped depend on how you resolve this conflict.

> ***The way through this conflict is to experience it and resolve it, and not avoid it in any way.***

As soon as you have smoked your last cigarette with the intention to quit, the conflict you feel could be deep and last for several hours. You may question yourself over and over again, asking yourself if you really do want to stop smoking, and whether this really is the right time to do it. You may spend hours trying to figure out a good excuse to justify smoking for just a little bit longer, or just one more . . .

Don't be surprised by this: it's all part of the process. The way through this conflict is to experience it and resolve it, and not avoid it in any way.

In order to resolve this conflict, you simply ask yourself this one, basic question: *Am I willing to accept my desire to smoke in order to stop smoking and stay stopped?* In other words, here you are feeling uncomfortable and unsatisfied because you want a cigarette but aren't smoking one; do you think it's worth it to you to feel this way in order to break free from a life of smoking?

Out of Sight, but Not Out of Mind

Some people avoid resolving this conflict by ignoring their desire and quite often feel confident that they have conquered their addiction. One of the more unhelpful things about repression is that, at the time you use it, it appears to be effective, and is therefore rarely perceived as being a problem.

You can see from your own experience that it is a problem, though, if you have ever stopped before. The first cigarette you smoked when you went back to smoking was preceded by a desire to smoke, even though you may have only been dimly aware of that desire at the time.

James, who attended a course of mine, gives us an example. He told me that at his last attempt, three years ago, he decided to stop smoking at the same time that he was going to redecorate his house. In other words, his strategy was to avoid as much of the difficulty of stopping smoking as he could by keeping busy painting and hanging paper.

He threw his cigarettes away and got rid of anything that might remind him of the smoker he used to be. The plan appeared to work and he managed to stop smoking with very little difficulty. He stayed stopped for a month, with smoking totally forgotten, until something happened that took him by surprise.

He told me that he was at the station where he commuted to work each day and went to the kiosk where he always used to buy his cigarettes. He asked for chewing gum, but the man behind the counter, recognising him, handed him his usual packet of cigarettes.

James took them, paid for them, opened the packet, took out a cigarette, lit it and was halfway through smoking it before he realised what he was doing. He was simply not aware of the desire to smoke that was guiding his actions. When he realised he was smoking he felt devastated, but the damage was already done: he had gone back to smoking again, and was soon smoking his usual number of cigarettes every day.

When you stop smoking by avoiding your desire to smoke, you have no way of controlling your automatic reaction once the desire finds a way to break through.

If James had spent some time during that month consciously dealing with his desire to smoke, then when he was given cigarettes by mistake at the station, he would have noticed there was a desire to smoke, and used The Outline (see page 116) to deal with it.

Learn to Induce the Desire

If, like James, you have stopped smoking in the past and not felt much of a desire, then you may well fall into the same pattern whenever you make an attempt to stop.

The best way to check yourself is by deliberately inducing your desire to smoke, so that you can retrain yourself to manage it and consciously accept it. *This might look as though you are making things more difficult for yourself, but in fact you are simply facing up to a difficulty that already exists.*

Inducing a desire to smoke is a conscious mental exercise. It means deliberately interrupting your thoughts about the other things in your life, and, with your cigarette packet in front of you, focusing on the feelings inside you of wanting to smoke.

There is a reason you are avoiding feeling your desire to smoke: you are no doubt afraid of it because you think it might make you smoke. You see it as an enemy, a nuisance and an unnecessary pain. When you deliberately induce it, you break down this negativity and fear, and turn the desire into something you have power over.

If you find inducing the desire difficult you will need to be creative. Watching other smokers light cigarettes can be helpful. Smelling your cigarettes in the packet or, if you used to make your own, rolling one up should produce the desire to smoke. For some people, imagining that they are smoking is the best way to connect with their desire to smoke. If you are really stuck in repression, buying a new pack of your favourite brand and taking the cellophane off may do the trick.

Sometimes people flirt with smoking, testing their limits to the point of putting a cigarette in their mouth and lighting a match. Obviously this is a dangerous game to play, and, by the way, a game that suggests you feel forbidden to smoke. It's not necessary to go this far: just looking at cigarettes in the pack should be enough for you to get in touch with your choice and desire to smoke them.

What you are doing is making a connection with the memory of your addiction: the memory stored in your mind that thinks smoking would be wonderful. Adverse thoughts will also be part of that memory, but don't use them to cancel out your desire because you need to work on accepting the desire, not denying it.

Some people will repress their desire to smoke from the moment they stop smoking. In that case, you will need to pause frequently, perhaps three or four times during each hour, and induce a desire you can really feel. It may take a while to work, but eventually you will feel a strong desire: an empty, uncomfortable sensation that you know would be relieved by smoking a cigarette.

For other people, repression only becomes a problem a few days or weeks after stopping. What happens is that the desire is so persistent at first that it is impossible to repress it, but as it fades in strength and frequency, it becomes increasingly possible to ignore it altogether.

After a few weeks of not smoking, you might need to induce your desire to smoke only once or twice a day. But it's important to do so because *it's only while you stay in touch with your desire to smoke that you can stay in control of it.*

Take advantage of familiar situations where you would have smoked, such as the end of a meal, as opportunities to induce your desire. Instead of jumping up from the table to get on with the washing-up, sit there for a while, as you would have done, let yourself feel your desire to smoke and think through The Outline.

Later on, your desire may only last a few seconds, but making a deliberate effort to acknowledge it by inducing it can make the difference between success and failure in the long term.

If you lead a very busy life, inducing your desire will be especially important. Busy people can stop smoking for days or weeks, barely aware of their desire to smoke in the background of their crowded minds. But just because you don't take the time to deal with it properly, the desire doesn't vanish; it keeps coming, like a nagging child demanding attention. Or it can suddenly and unexpectedly explode, perhaps at a time of crisis, and, because your conscious mind hasn't practised dealing with it, you can suddenly find yourself on the verge of smoking.

If you stop to induce a desire – and this only takes a few moments – you give your desire the attention it requires. As a result it becomes easy to live with and, most important of all, you are in control of it.

The Benefits of Inducing

It's difficult to describe how effective this is. At first glance, the idea of inducing your desire to smoke can seem perverse and masochistic: why tease yourself with temptation if what you really want to do is to never smoke again?

The reason is your memory. Just because the desire, and perhaps the cigarettes, is out of sight, it cannot be truly out of mind, because of your memory. By inducing, you learn to accept that part of your memory – the desire to smoke – whenever it becomes activated. If you use this technique, you will see for yourself how well it works.

When you first stop, you can expect to feel your desire to smoke at least as often as normal, in situations where you would have smoked. If you are in a situation where you never smoked – in a cinema, for example – then don't try to induce. But make sure you feel and manage your desire as soon as you leave that situation, if that's the time you would have smoked.

To begin with, the more you feel and experience your desire to smoke, the better. Inducing the desire is a very effective and powerful technique, and any time you use it – whether you think you are repressing or not – you will not be going wrong.

I have seen, through working with hundreds of smokers over many years, that those who use the technique of inducing their desire have an extremely high chance of success in the long term.

As time goes on, you will need to induce the desire less often but if you keep inducing it from time to time, your chances of staying stopped are excellent.

Why Welcome a Desire to Smoke?

Welcoming the desire to smoke is exactly the opposite of resisting it. When you welcome it you embrace and entertain it, becoming totally hospitable to this sensation of discomfort. *You make it your friend instead of your enemy.*

Each desire will inevitably pass in time: you don't get stuck in a permanent state of wanting to smoke. But the crucial move is to accept it while it's there. There are a number of reasons for this, and it's important to understand them in order to be able to live with something that is genuinely uncomfortable.

Your natural reaction will be to resist feeling uncomfortable: this is human nature. If you are too hot, you open a window. If there's a stone in your shoe, you take it out. Always you are attempting to maintain a state of comfort. This is an appropriate, self-correcting mechanism that helps you maintain a state of contented well-being, as much as you can.

With an addiction, however, this natural instinct for seeking comfort gets in the way. This is because, when it comes to breaking free from an addiction, the feeling of discomfort is absolutely the best thing to be experiencing, above all else.

Feeling the discomfort of an unsatisfied desire to smoke is your healing process, your recovery from addiction. Therefore, you need to deliberately intervene, to override your natural instincts, and remind yourself that, in this instance, discomfort is good for you.

It's good for you because while you are feeling it, you are not smoking. As a direct result of feeling the discomfort of your desire, you take control, and the quality of your life will improve in all kinds of ways. It may even, quite literally, save your life.

It's unlikely that you will welcome discomfort automatically. You need to consciously think this through to get yourself to see the value in it.

When you welcome your desire to smoke:

- You are far less likely to smoke unconsciously, without realising what you are doing, simply because you are able to consciously acknowledge its presence.
- You resolve the conflict you feel because you are saying, in no uncertain terms, that you'd rather feel this discomfort than spend the rest of your life smoking. Less conflict, less tension and anxiety.
- You overcome your fear of it, because when you welcome the desire nothing will make you smoke. This way you can quickly become confident about not smoking, in all kinds of situations and even under stress.
- You can see through the delusions that smoking will help you in some way – even, perhaps, that smoking is essential in some particular circumstance. You break your sense of dependency because you can see it more objectively as just another desire to smoke. Smoking simply satisfies it – nothing else.

- You release any tension (physical aches and nervous energy) you might otherwise build up in your fight against feeling the desire. It's like walking into a gale, and then changing direction so that the wind is behind you. When you welcome the discomfort, you are going along in the same direction. You can see that you have got a desire to smoke and you can be there with it and even relax with it.
- You let the desire 'burn off' like a kettle burning off steam. Avoiding and ignoring the desire doesn't do this, which is why it's essential to experience the feelings of desire when you have stopped smoking. It's not simply the passing of time that causes the desire to fade away. You heal the addiction through *feeling* your desire to smoke. *You feel it to heal it – and that's exactly how it diminishes in time.*

All you need to do is to identify the feeling of desire, pay attention to it for a moment, and say 'yes' to it and 'it's okay for me to feel this'. I don't mean to imply that you should enjoy it. Occasionally, people do tell me that they enjoy feeling their desire to smoke, but most people don't because it is genuinely uncomfortable. Welcoming it means you value it. *Welcoming it means you accept it unconditionally, and this gives you absolute control.*

You can see this discomfort as a payment, or a trade-off. By being willing to feel this temporarily uncomfortable sensation, you receive the benefits of not smoking. As a direct result of feeling the desire, you have more energy, greater self-respect, you feel cleaner and younger, you save lots of money and no longer live with the fear and guilt that smoking inevitably creates. Is it worth it? You decide!

I have worked with a few people who refuse to take this step. They stop smoking, but then they maintain that either way they go, they lose. Either they return to smoking, which they don't want to do. Or, from time to time, they feel their uncomfortable desire to smoke, which they don't want to do either. They hang on for a while, continuing to resent and resist their desire, even though it quickly diminishes to a couple of minutes of discomfort each day. Before long they return to smoking, with another failure behind them and even more resistance built into their minds.

The difference between success and failure in stopping smoking is not physical or chemical. It all comes down to your willingness to allow yourself to feel temporarily uncomfortable in order to gain the benefits of not smoking.

Your Freedom to Choose

If you do choose to smoke, of course, you return to smoking, satisfying your addictive desire with one cigarette after another. You reinforce your addiction, and run the risk of never stopping smoking again. If you remind yourself of your options in this way, by going through The Outline as much as you can, the alternative of accepting a few moments of discomfort will soon seem more attractive, and will continue to be the alternative you are most likely to choose.

It will help you to put the discomfort into the correct perspective. It is not torture. It is not a fate worse than death. It is just a temporary discomfort. It's intense at first, but it does fade. It's persistent at first, but it does become much less frequent. At first you may only just be able to accept the uncomfortable desire, but as it diminishes after the first couple of days, you can work towards welcoming it positively so that you fully resolve any conflict and resistance you may have towards it.

When you can be sure that you would rather feel your desire to smoke than live your life as a smoker, you have every chance of long-term success.

I have found that welcoming the desire is usually the very last thing people really understand about this technique, and some people never do! Those who do welcome it are the most successful in the long term, because of the simple fact that the desire to smoke rarely goes away completely, especially during the first year of not smoking.

IN OTHER WORDS: BARBARA

I started smoking at the age of 16, although it wasn't until I was about 19 that I became a heavy smoker, roughly 20 a day. Over the course of 20 years I smoked sometimes 30 cigarettes a day, and, am ashamed to say, continued puffing through both of my pregnancies. I tried to stop smoking, or cut down as much as I could, but to no avail.

To be quite honest, I never dreamed that I would be able to stop, but four years have passed now, and I feel so much better. My skin doesn't have that sort of yellowy look!

The most helpful thing that I learned from Full Stop was the technique of holding the cigarette packet during those first few days of giving up. I can remember ironing with one hand, while the other clutched the cherished cigarette packet. Even now I use the techniques in my mind to overcome the feeling of wanting to smoke.

The best thing about not smoking is feeling better, no more tenseness around the neck and shoulders, and not feeling reliant on something that is not natural. Also, the theatre and cinema outings are more enjoyable now. As a smoker I would be looking anxiously at my watch, waiting for the interval to arrive. The feeling of freedom from all of that is like a weight lifted from my shoulders.

The most difficult time I have experienced since stopping was when my father was critically ill, in intensive care. However, he fully recovered I'm glad to say, and by using the Full Stop method I managed to get through it as well!

This is the only positive way to stop smoking. You can do it, with determination and the knowledge of these techniques.

CHAPTER 12

Moments of Truth

It is in this whole process of meeting and solving problems that life has its meaning. Problems are the cutting edge that distinguishes between success and failure. Problems call forth our courage and our wisdom; indeed, they create our courage and our wisdom.

M. SCOTT PECK, *THE ROAD LESS TRAVELLED*

Because most people don't want to feel their desire to smoke after they have stopped, they often try to avoid any circumstance that has an association with smoking. They reorganise their lives as much as they can, so that they will be faced with temptation as little as possible.

If someone goes to a particular pub regularly, then they avoid the pub when they stop smoking, staying home in the evenings instead. If they used to smoke at work, they might decide to stop smoking while they are away on holiday, to avoid facing their working day without a cigarette.

Parties, friends who smoke, coffee breaks, demanding work and long journeys are all typical situations that ex-smokers fear and often go to great lengths to avoid during the first weeks, and even months, of not smoking. And you may find that you consider this path to some extent.

The most obvious problem with this kind of strategy is that it is totally impractical to try to avoid all the situations that may trigger a strong desire to smoke. You simply cannot avoid everything that might be stressful, upsetting, enjoyable, demanding, social or boring, to name just a few examples, unless you just stop living.

But even if you do manage to eliminate most of these situations from your life, what is it that you are really avoiding? It's not the situation. You have coped with those countless times and have no special fear of them. What you are trying to avoid, of course, is the desire to smoke you know you will face.

While following this strategy of avoidance might appear to help you with stopping smoking initially, it certainly won't help you to stay stopped. It's actually one of the biggest factors that explains why people don't stay stopped.

When you deliberately avoid the potentially more difficult situations, what you are really doing is accepting your desire to smoke only *conditionally*. You establish in your mind that you will accept your desire to smoke, and thereby stay stopped, *provided* you are not with any smokers. Or *provided* you're sober. You'll do it *provided* you're not upset. Or *provided* you're not bored, tired or under any stress. And above all, *provided* your desire to smoke is not too intense.

Unfortunately, your addiction doesn't strike bargains. And if you ever try to make a compromise with it, you end up the loser.

The desire to smoke will continue to reappear from time to time in all kinds of circumstances, long after you have stopped smoking. This is inevitable. The only strategy that is going to keep you from smoking, in the long term, is for you to be willing to accept feeling it from time to time, no matter where you are and no matter what is going on.

The way to stop smoking and stay stopped for good is to come to an unconditional acceptance of your addictive desire to smoke – and to do it as soon as possible after you have stopped smoking.

In certain circumstances your desire to smoke will be more intense and persistent. These are the circumstances where you have developed a stronger dependency on smoking. It's understandable that you will be concerned about whether you will get through them without smoking. What will make all the difference is how you cope with this fear, right from the beginning.

Remember from Chapter 5 that you can stop worrying about an approaching situation by staying in the present. You can only manage your desire to smoke at the time you are actually feeling it, so don't even try to predict what you will do. If you avoid the situation, however, you reinforce your fear by giving it more credibility.

If you avoid a difficult or tempting situation, you cannot possibly break from your dependency. You can only do this by going into each situation, learning how to handle it without smoking, and dealing with your desire to smoke at the time.

Does this sound like needless torture? It's not. What would really be needless torture would be living in fear of being overwhelmed one day by an intense desire to smoke. Needless torture would be trying to make changes in yourself and your life in the hope that you will eliminate your inevitable desire. *Needless torture is stopping smoking, but not doing anything to break your psychological dependency, and so going back to smoking over and over again.*

Keep to Your Routines

First of all, you need to know whether or not you are about to avoid anything when you stop smoking. In order to do this, just ask yourself: *Would I be doing this if I hadn't stopped smoking?* For the first couple of weeks, as much as possible, stay with all your familiar routines.

Social situations. Go to the pub or to parties just as often as you always have done. Be there as you usually would, with a drink in your hand and everyone smoking around you. Think through The Outline (see page 116) to yourself and make private choices to accept your desire, because as far as you're concerned, at least for now, you prefer to be someone who doesn't smoke.

Daily routines. Follow all your normal routines as a smoker, exactly as you used to do. Notice any changes you might be thinking of making, however innocent or well-intentioned they appear to be.

Let's say that you feel like taking your dog for a walk one evening, a day or two after you've stopped smoking. Ask yourself what you would be doing if you hadn't stopped smoking. If you normally take your dog for a walk each evening, then go ahead and do it.

If, however, you don't, then it's likely you are in fact wanting to avoid something: perhaps a half-hour of sitting around with not much to do before dinner? You would have been smoking, and your sudden interest in your dog's exercise is really nothing more than your avoidance of your desire to smoke.

Places you smoked. Don't avoid the places where you used to smoke – your favourite chair, desk, kitchen table. If your house is a no-smoking zone, you may have stepped out to the garden whenever you wanted to smoke. To begin with, take your usual trips to the garden, with your cigarettes, and make your choice to accept your desire to smoke there.

At work. If you used to smoke at work, your first working day after you have stopped smoking can be quite a challenge, because you may well have the kind of job where demands are constantly being made on your attention.

It's realistic to assume that you might not be working at your best for the first few days, because of the constant distraction of wanting to smoke. But the more you take time to deal with your desire to smoke, the sooner things will get better.

By far the most effective approach is to pause, mentally, at least a couple of times during an hour, and focus directly on your desire and deal with it by thinking through The Outline.

This doesn't make the desire go away: it's not supposed to. But when you remind yourself of your choices and make a clear choice to accept or even welcome the desire, then you will find that you can return your attention to your work and continue for a bit longer.

If your work is very hectic, you may need to plan special strategies so you can take this personal time with your own mind. You could pretend you are reading something for a few moments, or, as a last resort, take yourself off to the toilet.

You probably have special routines at work when you would go to a particular place to light up a cigarette. It might be someone else's office, a smoking room or outside the back door. For at least the first week, make sure you don't avoid any of these. Take as many breaks as you normally would, go to those same places, take your cigarettes with you, and deal with your desire to smoke!

Some people claim they are just too busy to do this, or that their work is too important and too demanding to spend so much time thinking about smoking. It's a matter of choosing to make stopping smoking a number one priority for a while, and in the long run your work will benefit.

Many people make the fundamental mistake of thinking that if they hang on long enough without smoking, things will improve by themselves.

An addicted smoker is a less-efficient worker: buying and smoking cigarettes takes up time, you can get distracted during meetings where you are not allowed to smoke, you get more tired and stressed because of your smoking, and need more time off work due to smoking-related illness.[1]

If you decide you are too busy to spend any time dealing with your desire to smoke, it might be more honest for you to admit that it's really because you just don't want to bother.

Many people make the fundamental mistake of thinking that if they hang on long enough without smoking, things will improve by themselves. I wish it were true, and I should think that a great many relapsed smokers do too. What happens if you keep pushing your desire to smoke to one side is that you can end up feeling tense, frustrated and disorientated. Also, you might be able to avoid feeling your desire all day at work, but get hit with it on your way home. Or you might be able to ignore it for a week or two, but then return to smoking at the very first crisis that comes along.

Concentrating. A common result of not dealing with the desire is that you become unable to concentrate properly on anything at all, and the longer you avoid dealing with this, the longer your lack of concentration will go on, continuing for weeks and even months. Your work may require you to concentrate on writing, for example, and if you simply avoid doing the work, putting it off until you feel more like tackling it, you will end up reinforcing the delusion that you actually can't work without smoking! Which is the perfect 'rational' excuse to resume doing it . . .

The way to break this delusion is to sit down to write as usual, and expect to feel your desire to smoke. The association between writing and smoking has been made, so the desire will be there as an automatic reflex. Focus your attention on the desire and deal with it, deliberately and carefully, by thinking through The Outline, making a clear choice to acknowledge it, and accept it. Then, without fighting the desire, bring your attention back to what you are doing.

This will slow you down a bit at first, but even if you write just a little without smoking to begin with, you are proving to yourself, gradually, that your beliefs about your dependency are completely fictitious. It's only when you've discovered that you really can write without smoking that you will be likely to stay stopped, and you can only do that by going ahead and writing, even though it may look impossible at first. You are re-educating yourself, and at first it might even seem like you are learning to write all over again.

I have worked with a number of professional writers who, through exactly the same process, have successfully stayed stopped and also learned to continue to write. One novelist client told me that his main problem was more with his fear that he wouldn't be able to write without smoking.

As soon as he had written the first piece that looked okay, he felt much more confident, and he has never looked back. Now he is busy with a new novel, and he finds he still occasionally gets the desire to smoke, particularly when he is looking for inspiration. The key for him is in knowing that the inspiration will come anyway, without the cigarettes.

If you take other drugs. One of the situations most frequently avoided when people stop smoking is that of drinking alcohol. Your fear (as if I needed to tell you) is that you will not be able to be in control of yourself if you are intoxicated.

As someone who smoked while drinking you will undoubtedly experience a strong desire to smoke whenever you drink, especially at first. But this is nothing more than the same desire that has been triggered in your mind by the conditioned association you created over the years. And you are just as capable of thinking through The Outline and making a choice to accept it as you are when you are sober.

If you usually drink alcohol, don't avoid it at all when you stop smoking. Drink as you normally would; drink the same amounts in the same situations, and deal with the desire to smoke as it comes along, in the normal way.

You are still capable of managing your desire to smoke, even if you have had a few drinks. Even after a few, you can still set your own limits to your behaviour. If you know you can draw the line when you want to about other things when you are drunk, like jumping into bed with anyone you fancy, or driving your car, then you can also choose to be in control of whether or not you smoke a cigarette, if you want to.

It's probably not a good idea to get extremely drunk for the first day or two after you have stopped smoking. In fact, if you do, it's more likely to be a problem of substitution (see

Chapter 13). But, as with other avoidances, it's going to be much better for you to overcome your fears as soon as possible and face that intense desire to smoke the first time you sit down with a glass of beer or a bottle of wine.

This also applies to taking 'recreational' drugs, such as cannabis or cocaine. Again, the association with smoking cigarettes is strong, but the same process applies: don't avoid it, for the same reasons, and expect and accept your desire to smoke cigarettes, which will be intense at first.

I'm not encouraging or advocating the use of drugs: the two just mentioned are illegal, and, to varying degrees, addictive and dangerous as well. What I am saying is that if you usually take these drugs, don't stop taking them at the same time as you stop smoking cigarettes. This adds up to an avoidance of the desire to smoke cigarettes, as far as dealing with your addiction to nicotine is concerned.

You may or may not be addicted to other drugs and you may or may not want to stop taking them later on, but this is another matter. When you stop smoking, it's important to deal with that one drug: nicotine. Then, whatever other drugs you may be taking, you will find you are able to stay off nicotine, because you have dealt with it as a separate issue.

When it comes to cannabis, it's easy to get confused, for two reasons. One is that it is usually smoked like a cigarette. But this doesn't mean that it is a cigarette, as long as it doesn't have any tobacco (nicotine) with it. You inhale its smoke into your lungs but you are still not absorbing nicotine.

The complication is that cannabis is often mixed and smoked together with tobacco. It's important to be very clear about this. If you make a choice to smoke tobacco together with cannabis, then you are back to your old nicotine addiction again, and you will inevitably return to smoking cigarettes. Tobacco is by far the more addictive drug of the two, and smoking even a puff of a joint containing tobacco will take you back to smoking cigarettes on a regular basis.

At the same time, *it's essential that you do not substitute any other drugs for cigarettes in the process of stopping smoking.* In other words, be careful not to increase your use of other substances at the time you stop smoking. Chapter 13 will explain how.

There are many people who use drugs, and have every intention of continuing to use them. But it's completely unnecessary to be stuck with smoking tobacco as well.

If this applies to you, understand that you can stop smoking tobacco and stay in control of your addiction to nicotine, if you use this technique with honesty and care. And you can use what you have learned to help deal with other addictions, if you want to, later on.

Continue to Deal with the Desire

During your first week of not smoking, you will start to feel your desire to smoke less often. As it diminishes, it will still be important to keep dealing with it as much as possible. Even many weeks after stopping smoking, when you may only feel your desire once or twice a day, managing the desire will make the crucial difference as to whether you stay stopped or not.

By advising you not to avoid anything, I do not mean you should never make any changes in your routines. After the first two weeks, go ahead and make any changes you want. It's just that the first time you encounter situations in which you smoked, you will probably feel a stronger desire to smoke.

It Gets Easier

Although it can certainly seem more difficult at first, facing all these situations from the very beginning, instead of avoiding them, actually makes things much easier for you in the long run.

The most challenging times can be the most ordinary: sitting at your kitchen table, talking on the phone, driving your car. When you have faced these things once without smoking, then the next time you are in that situation, it will be much easier for you to deal with. And the reason it is easier is because you have created a new memory: a memory of being in that situation without smoking, perhaps for the first time in years. You did it, you survived, and you didn't smoke. And it will be even easier the next time, because the desire will be that bit less intense and that bit less persistent, and because smoking will seem that bit less necessary.

Without any warning, you walk into an argument, or there's an accident and, inevitably, there's also an intense desire to smoke.

Each time you face the situation, and the resulting desire to smoke, you reaffirm to yourself that you would rather accept feeling the desire than return to smoking. *The more often you do this when you first stop smoking, the greater your chances of success in the long term and the sooner you will break free from your dependency.*

Many people tell me that the circumstances they were most concerned about usually turned out to be much easier than they had feared. It's actually the surprises that are hardest to handle, precisely because they cannot be anticipated.

Suddenly, without any warning, you walk into an argument, or there's an accident and, inevitably, there's also an intense desire to smoke. There is no way you can avoid these things happening in your life, but if you have been practising dealing with your desire to smoke anyway, you will see your desire to smoke at times of upset as nothing more than just another desire to smoke for you to make a choice about.

Temptations exist, and you will be faced with one sooner or later. While you are trying to avoid the inevitable desire to smoke, you are not developing an acceptance of it. You cannot do both, and unless you overcome your fear of your desire to smoke, and learn to accept and manage it – regardless of whatever situation you are in – you are very likely to return to smoking eventually.

Before attending a course with me, a client named Marianne used to stop smoking regularly, at least twice a year, while staying at a health farm.

She told me that at these times she was very eager to stop smoking and that stopping seemed effortless. Each time she stopped she fully intended to stay stopped, and was genuinely puzzled by her repeated relapses back into smoking, either on her return home, or very soon after.

What Marianne needed to learn was that, although she was highly motivated to stop smoking, without training her mind to manage her desire to smoke (repressed during her health farm visits), she had no way to turn her motivation into real success.

When she learned this technique, she started to face and take control of her addiction in her normal routines, and at the time of writing has stayed stopped over 10 months, which is very much longer than she ever did before.

IN OTHER WORDS: TIM

In truth I no longer believed that I could stop, even if I had really wanted to. So most of the time I did not let myself admit that I wanted to, which made it easier to live with myself.

But there were times when, above all, the fear of the consequences would get to me and I would try almost anything to stop myself wanting a cigarette. Because I associated smoking with all the unhealthy things in my life, I would turn instead to all the things that I associated with health and fitness. So I would go for long, invigorating walks, or take up swimming regularly; I would cycle to work and make plans to join a gym and get myself super fit. I would cut down on alcohol, give up drinking coffee, which I've always accompanied with at least one cigarette, and drink mineral water instead. Altogether I devised a punitively puritanical regime.

Such resolutions were inevitably ill-fated. Around every corner lurked the demon I was running away from. I would say to myself: 'Let me be fit and healthy, but let me first have a cigarette!'

And then the truth dawned – or rather it was pointed out to me. That there was no necessary connection between all these things. That stopping smoking was simply about stopping smoking: it was not about taking up anything else. All I needed to do was acknowledge that I wanted to smoke, that I was quite free to do so, and at the same time I didn't have to just at the moment.

What I had seen as an overpowering menace that had left me feeling defeated and very feeble was reduced at a stroke to simple, manageable proportions.

CHAPTER 13

You Don't Have to Gain Weight

The objects of desire are like salt water. The more we enjoy them the more our craving will increase.

TIBETAN BUDDHIST SAYING

At some time in the process of stopping smoking you will most likely experience, probably quite briefly, a thrill at the thought of success. Even before you've stopped there may be a moment when you begin to believe that stopping really is possible for you, and you feel excited with hope. More likely it will be after you've stopped, when you start to experience the undeniable reality of the fact that you're not smoking.

This thrill of success can be subtle because it's usually such a fleeting feeling, yet also extremely powerful because it's so life-affirming. You may find you react to it in one of two ways.

One is to ride with it and say 'yes' to it. Yes, this is wonderful; yes, I'm wonderful for stopping smoking; yes, life is wonderful when things like this happen. There is no problem with this reaction, provided you remember you can only stay stopped for each moment as it comes; it's *always* 'so far, so good . . .'

The other reaction to success is the one that can create problems, because it can knock you off balance. This reaction happens to people who find it difficult to accept success like this in their lives because they have low self-esteem.

The best way to explain this is to refer you to a book called *The Six Pillars of Self-Esteem* by Dr Nathaniel Branden (published in the USA by Bantam Press). I have adapted the following passage from this book, and present it here with kind permission from the author:

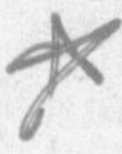

> Self-esteem – whether it's high or low – tends to be a generator of self-fulfilling prophecies. With high self-esteem, we are more likely to persist in the face of difficulties. With low self-esteem, we are more likely to give up or go through the motions of trying without really giving our best. Either way, our view of ourselves will be reinforced.
>
> But what happens if we do succeed at something, even though we have low self-esteem? Then our 'knowledge' about ourselves (e.g. 'I'm hopeless') doesn't match up with the facts (e.g. successfully stopping smoking) and we can begin to feel anxious, as if there is something dreadfully wrong.
>
> If our 'knowledge' is never questioned, it is the facts that may have to be altered. Guided unconsciously by the deepest logic of our self-concept, we get rid of the anxiety by getting rid of the success: hence self-sabotage. This is the basic pattern of self-destruction: if I 'know' my fate is to be unhappy and unsuccessful, I must not allow reality to confuse me with too much happiness and success.
>
> People sabotage themselves at the height of their success all the time. They do so when success clashes

> with their implicit beliefs about what is appropriate to them. It is frightening to be flung beyond the limits of one's idea of who one is. If a self-concept cannot accommodate a given level of success, and if the self-concept does not change, that person may find some way to sabotage their success.
>
> Their success activates internal voices saying: 'I don't deserve this' or 'it will never last' or 'my life is not like this' or 'people will be envious and hate me' or 'nobody else is happy, so why should I be?' We need to confront those destructive voices, not run from them. What is required for many of us is the courage to tolerate success without self-sabotage, until such time as we lose our fear of it and realise that it will not destroy us – and need not disappear.

Of course, the most direct way to sabotage your success at stopping smoking is to return to smoking, but there's another road many people take, and that is to eat food instead of smoking cigarettes. For example, after you stop smoking you eat a biscuit or two with a cup of coffee where before you would have had a cigarette. Or you have a dessert after a meal where before you ended your meals by smoking. So instead of smoking, you are eating something.

This sabotages your success in two ways. First, it leads to weight gain, so any sense of success from having stopped smoking tends to get cancelled out by misery over the extra pounds.

But the substitution of food also has a sabotaging effect on your smoking addiction. This is because when you eat food instead of smoking cigarettes you are still feeding your addictive desire, so it's almost as if you are still smoking. Smoking satisfies your desire to smoke with a cigarette.

Substituting food satisfies your desire to smoke with something to eat. In a way, *you are smoking food.*

The extra calories you consume add up to extra pounds, but substitution isn't just a problem with weight. Substituting anything for a cigarette, whether it contains calories or not, has a damaging effect because every time you satisfy any addictive desire, you reinforce and strengthen it. The tricky thing about all this is that you may end up not with a stronger desire to smoke, but with a stronger desire to eat.

You see, *if you reinforce your desire to smoke by eating, that desire will very rapidly change itself into an addictive desire to eat.*

Here's an example of how this happens. Let's say that for the first day or two after stopping smoking you really feel like a cigarette with your mid-morning cup of coffee because that's when you used to smoke. So you decide to eat a bar of chocolate as a substitute for the cigarette. You think: 'I want a cigarette, but I've stopped smoking, so I'll have a chocolate bar.' But very soon – because the addiction can adapt very quickly – you are just thinking: 'I want some chocolate.' You've trained yourself to expect a snack when before you expected a cigarette. You've created an increased, addictive appetite.

This can be a very seductive trap, because when you substitute food, stopping smoking can seem relatively easy. This is because you don't want to smoke all that much. Your desire to smoke diminishes very rapidly and can even be gone entirely after a few days if you substitute enough.

What little desire to smoke you do feel, you find you can easily accept, but you are only accepting what you are aware of, which is merely the tip of the iceberg. Most of your desire to smoke is appearing as an addictive desire to eat. You experience a brief and acceptable desire to smoke, but also a persistent addictive hunger, which you are satisfying.

Please note that the example of the chocolate as the mid-morning snack is just that: one example. When people substitute food, they don't substitute just once, or in just one situation. *They train themselves to desire food where before they desired cigarettes.* So the addictive desire to eat will occur many times during the day, every day. If the way you respond to it is to feed it, you will of course gain weight.

You will be feeding an insatiable appetite, because the action of feeding this appetite keeps it alive.

Weight gain may be the most obvious problem with feeding an increased appetite, but the really insidious result of substitution is that while you are substituting, you are not working towards gaining a genuine acceptance of your desire to smoke. You are not making choices to accept your desire to smoke; you are feeding it, trying to satisfy it.

And you will be feeding an insatiable appetite, because the action of feeding this appetite keeps it alive. As your addictive appetite gets larger and larger, so do you.

Finally, you may return to smoking because you don't know any other way to stop yourself from eating so much.

How to Break the Cycle

This depressing cycle from smoking to overeating and back to smoking again may be an all-too-familiar one for you. For many smokers, staying stopped for good will only be realistic when a way can be found to control the substitution of food for cigarettes. The answer lies, once again, in The Outline and in your acceptance of your addictive desires.

Here are four simple steps for you to use. My advice is for you to be very careful about this for the first few weeks after you have stopped smoking. *The longer you go without substituting food, the less likely you are to start.* Face up to the difficulty in the beginning and things will get easier as you go on.

1 *Notice what you eat and drink.* First of all, it's essential to become aware of any potential substitutions. If you are not aware that you are just about to substitute, you can do nothing to control it.

This may seem obvious, but it is one of the most common problems. Eating is an ordinary daily activity, and it's very, very easy to gradually increase amounts without realising what you are doing. This is especially likely to happen if you are not a weight-watching, calorie-counting kind of eater in the first place. After you stop smoking, you may need to become much more aware of your eating, and not just go ahead and eat automatically every time you feel like it.

2 *Ask yourself: would I be doing this if I hadn't stopped smoking?* It's very possible that you don't feel a desire to smoke; you feel hungry or perhaps you just fancy something to eat. So you need to find out first of all if what you are about to eat is a substitution for smoking or not. There is really only one way to tell if you are about to substitute, and that is to ask yourself, before you eat or drink anything, whether or not it's something you would have consumed when you were a smoker.

If it's something you usually eat at this time and place, then go ahead and eat it. If it isn't, then realise that what you have is an addictive desire – a desire to smoke in disguise. If you identify it, it will be possible for you to deal with it.

3 *If in doubt, play it safe.* If you are not sure whether or not you would have eaten a particular thing at a particular time as a smoker, it's best to err on the safe side and assume it's a substitution.

For example, you may get to the end of a meal and feel like some ice-cream. You ask yourself if you would have had ice-cream when you were smoking and you honestly don't know. Some days you had ice-cream after dinner and some days you didn't, and you have no way of knowing whether today is the day you would have had it.

My advice is for you to skip the ice-cream. The worst thing that will happen is that you pass on something you might possibly have eaten. The best thing that will happen is that *you train yourself not to accept food as an alternative way of satisfying your desire to smoke.* If you establish this in the early days after stopping smoking, it will get easier in time.

4 *Use The Outline* (see page 116). This step is vital! Don't forget that when you are about to substitute some food for a cigarette, you are experiencing your addictive desire to smoke.

First, see if you can get in touch with the desire to smoke that is lurking behind your desire to eat. Take out a pack of cigarettes, and try to induce your desire to smoke. You may feel it as a desire to smoke, but whether you do or whether it just stays as a desire to eat, go through The Outline and make your choice.

It's crucial to stick to what you normally eat *because the addictive desire to eat and the addictive desire to smoke can be difficult to tell apart.* They can both be experienced as:

- a thought
- wanting something in your mouth
- wanting something to do with your hands
- emptiness, 'butterflies' or tension in your stomach.

Any addictive desire feels like an uncomfortable void that wants to be filled. Your addictive desire to eat can feel like hunger, an increased appetite and/or greater attraction to food of all kinds.

Any addictive desire feels like an uncomfortable void that wants to be filled.

It can also be experienced as thirst. Substitution of coffee can result in nervous anxiety, especially as caffeine has more of an effect on you without nicotine in your system. Substitution of alcohol creates its own problems, including weight gain. And remember from Chapter 12 that it is just as problematic to substitute other drugs. The principles described in this chapter can be applied to any potential substitution for cigarettes. I'm concentrating on the substitution of food because it's by far the most common.

People often think of substitution as manic bingeing. It can be, but it is far more frequently subtle and sporadic. It can be a few biscuits here, and a bar of chocolate there, and an extra helping of casserole at dinner . . . and two stones later you are seriously considering returning to smoking.

When you first stop smoking, expect to have an increased interest in food. Expect to have more of an appetite, *especially wanting to go on eating at the end of a meal.*

Expect to want more meals, more snacks and larger amounts.

What will make all the difference is whether you feed this extra desire to eat or whether you make choices to accept it. When you feed it, you reinforce it. You satisfy it for the present time, but it comes back again later and rapidly becomes a persistent addictive hunger, integrated into your daily life.

If you simply accept it, let yourself feel it and don't try to get rid of it at all, the addictive hunger will begin to diminish after a day or two and will become increasingly easier to deal with. Then – *and only then* – you break the connection between smoking and eating. You will be able to do that if you are aware of what is really going on.

Myths About Smoking and Weight

'*Nicotine suppresses my hunger.*' First of all, it will help us to be clear about what kind of hunger we are talking about. Many people rarely feel a *genuine* hunger, a sign of a natural and appropriate need for nourishment. Instead, they feed and encourage an *addictive* hunger, over and above their real nutritional needs. Just as the addictive desire to smoke is created by making choice after choice to smoke, so the addictive desire to eat (excess appetite) is created by making choice after choice to overeat.

What's very helpful to know is that it can be *virtually impossible to tell these two kinds of hunger apart*, especially for those who overeat a lot. Like the desire to smoke, natural and addictive appetites are both experienced as thoughts (in the mind) and as sensations (in the body, especially the mouth and stomach).

People who are overweight may rarely feel their natural hunger, if at all. They usually feed their addictive hunger before it becomes a natural hunger. Some people even fear natural hunger, so eat more food than they need in order to keep it at bay.

The generally accepted myth is that nicotine represses hunger, yet research has shown that nicotine replacement products don't alleviate hunger at all during withdrawal from smoking.[1]

The reason for this is that the extra hunger people feel when they stop smoking is not a genuine need for nutrition, but an addictive hunger. Natural hunger alone is very easy and even pleasant to live with for reasonable periods of time. It comes and goes regardless of whether you smoke or not, and only becomes a problem if you wait so long before you eat that you become weak or faint through lack of necessary nourishment.

When someone thinks that nicotine is suppressing their hunger, what is usually happening is that they are satisfying their addictive hunger with addictive smoking.

One final note about natural hunger. People with stomach acidity or stomach ulcers may well find that natural hunger is painful, and not at all pleasant to live with. If this is the case for you, stopping smoking is the best step you can take, as smoking is a major cause of these problems.

'My metabolism has changed since I stopped smoking.' Research has shown that metabolism speeds up a little when a person first starts to smoke, but that the body soon adapts to this. This means that the effect wears off, so that smokers are not in any better position than those who don't smoke. In fact, after years of smoking, smokers are in a far worse position as far as metabolic rate is concerned. This is why.

Your base metabolic rate is whatever energy it takes for you to simply stay alive: it's measured as how fast your body burns up calories when you are at rest. As you may know, some people have a faster metabolism than others. But why? The key factor is the amount of lean muscle mass on your body. The more lean muscle mass you have, the more calories you burn, and as a result, the higher your metabolic rate. So if you think you are someone who has a slow metabolism, that's the reason: you have lost some amount of lean muscle mass over the years. This is extremely common, especially for smokers.

The problem is that smoking greatly impairs your body's ability to maintain its lean mass. This is why, over time, a smoker's metabolic rate falls faster than that of a non-smoker.

A study conducted at Glasgow University, looking at the smoking habits of more than 1,000 young women, found that *the smokers were more likely to put on weight.* Not only were the smokers heavier, but they also had larger waist measurements. The cause of this was the lean muscle mass damage caused by smoking.[2]

So why, you might ask, is it so widely believed that metabolism slows down when a smoker quits? By far the greatest culprit in gaining weight lies in the substitution of food and drink for cigarettes. If your metabolic rate is low due to years of smoking, you will be especially prone to weight gain with even the smallest increase in caloric intake.

If your weight is important to you, my advice is to stop smoking as soon as possible. Then get to work on building and maintaining your lean muscle mass. It's well known that any kind of exercise achieves this; it's less well known that the same result comes from eating plenty of fresh fruit and vegetables.

'I know my metabolism has changed because I'm constipated.' But constipation isn't caused by changes in your metabolism, which is simply the rate at which your body burns calories.

Constipation, though, can certainly leave you feeling bloated and miserable, and it can be wise to take steps to avoid this problem. First, let's see why it happens.

A healthy human colon contains beneficial bacteria, designed to complete the digestion process. Much of this bacteria, vital to our health, is killed off by chemical residues in our food, antibiotics and steroids. It is also killed by the poison nicotine. This would lead to constipation for the smoker, but nicotine also has the effect of artificially stimulating the bowel, so the problem is not discovered until the smoker stops smoking.

Good, effective remedies for constipation are available, and you don't have to settle for old-fashioned laxatives, which can be rather harsh. You can ask for your doctor's advice, take probiotic supplements (e.g. *Lactobacillus acidophilus*) to replenish the bacteria or ask at a good health food shop.

Watch Out for the Excuses

'I have a healthy appetite when I stop smoking.' It's true that you may have improved senses of taste and smell after you stop smoking. But just because food tastes better, that doesn't mean you have to eat larger amounts!

You do not have a 'healthy appetite': you have an addictive appetite. There is no valid need to consume more food just because you have stopped smoking. If anything, you need less food, because smoking depletes vitamins.

There are some smokers who don't eat enough, and as a result are underweight. In this case, a genuinely healthy appetite will normally be restored after stopping smoking, but it's still wise to be very careful about substitution in the form of addictive eating.

'*At least I'm not smoking.*' This is a very common way to rationalise substitution; eating instead of smoking yourself to death can seem the lesser of two evils. But substitution is a short-term 'solution' that creates long-term difficulties. And one of those long-term difficulties can be a return to smoking, because of uncontrollable weight gain, and because the repressed desire to smoke hasn't been dealt with and accepted.

'*I know I'm not substituting, because my clothes still fit me.*' It depends a great deal on you and your size and style of clothes, but it is possible to put on as much as a stone before you notice it. Unfortunately, many people only get serious about dealing with their substitution problem *after* they've got upset about their weight gain.

This makes the whole problem more drawn out, and if you do take this path, expect to feel a stronger and more frequent desire to smoke whenever you do stop substituting, since when you cut back on your eating it will no longer stay repressed.

'*I'll take the weight off later.*' In case you don't know this, it's actually a lot easier not to put the weight on in the first place. Maintaining weight is tough enough for most of us: losing it is a very slow business.

'*I smoke to control my addictive overeating.*' If this is how you see things, it will be helpful for you to identify which addictive behaviour you prefer, which one is your 'drug of choice'. The way you do this is to ask yourself: if you had just enough food to keep you alive, and the option of an unlimited supply of only *one* addiction, with no hazardous consequences, what would it be? For many smokers the answer would clearly be cigarettes, while for others it would be food.

If you answered the latter, you see yourself more as an addictive overeater who smokes in order to control their eating, rather than as a smoker who turns to food in an attempt to stop smoking. Maybe the only reason you smoke at all is because you don't know any other way to stop yourself from eating so much.

Maybe the only reason you smoke at all is because you don't know any other way to stop yourself from eating so much.

Addictive eating has a great deal in common with addictive smoking, and many of the principles explained in this book apply equally to both. I suggest you take a look at my book on this, *Eating Less: Say Goodbye to Overeating*. See page 195 for more details.

This book will help you to stop smoking, which is your first step. When you stop smoking, don't even try to eliminate the addictive overeating you may already do: just make sure it doesn't increase, for any reason, as a substitution for smoking.

One thing you can be sure of is that you can never properly deal with your addiction to food while you are still smoking. You create and maintain a powerful addiction to nicotine and you never learn how to really control your addictive desire for food. After many years of smoking, when both addictions are well established, smoking often becomes a less and less effective way to control addictive overeating: hence, overweight smokers.

'I'm substituting, but I know I'm doing it.' I've often heard this from clients who suppose that consciously choosing to substitute somehow eliminates any problems. It doesn't.

Common Questions

'Whenever I eat it seems I satisfy my desire to smoke. Am I substituting?' When you first stop smoking, your desire to smoke will be quite persistent, so it's entirely possible that you will feel as if you are satisfying it any time you eat or drink anything at all.

This is why it's so helpful to identify substitutions with the question: *Would I be doing this if I hadn't stopped smoking?* So you don't ask yourself if you are hungry, because you may have a false hunger that is really a desire to smoke, or you may have a real hunger because it's lunchtime. You don't ask yourself if you really want to eat or if you really want to smoke, because you may want either one or both at the same time.

Your desire to smoke may well disappear while you are eating, just as it may disappear while you are playing tennis, for example. This is not a substitution if it's what you normally do. Just make sure you manage your desire to smoke if it reappears, as it is likely to do, when you finish your meal or activity.

'Is it okay to substitute cinnamon sticks, chewing gum or water?' Substitution is not just a potential weight problem: it's the choice to feed your desire to smoke, instead of accepting it. The desire to smoke may or may not get repressed as a result, but the act of substituting always reinforces your addictive desire to smoke and/or eat.

It's a mistake to think you can substitute selectively. If you begin to substitute, even a cup of tea or a piece of fruit, you establish substitution as an alternative you are going to take. Then you will have an increased addictive desire to eat which you will want to satisfy with whatever food is available at the time, whether you happen to be at a salad bar or in a bakery. This is especially true if you have addictive eating patterns anyway.

'*Shouldn't I exercise more after I've stopped smoking, to increase my metabolism/keep my weight down/take care of constipation?*' Even if you make a change like this for the very best reasons, there are three ways in which this can sabotage your process of stopping smoking.

First, your ability to stay stopped easily becomes dependent on your new routine. In order to be somebody who doesn't smoke, you need to be fit, energetic and generally on top of things. As soon as you don't feel quite so motivated and positive, you are more likely to return to smoking.

Second, the time you take exercising may well be time you would have spent smoking. This means you avoid feeling and managing your desire to smoke at that time. You will find that it makes all the difference if you use The Outline at every opportunity, especially to begin with so that you can retrain your mind.

Third, if you increase your exercise it's easier to justify substituting food, because you can tell yourself that weight won't become a problem. But remember, substitution isn't just a weight problem, it's a feeding-your-addictive-desire problem.

I recommend you keep to all your normal routines for at least two weeks after stopping.

'For years I've been substituting mints for cigarettes during the day because I'm not allowed to smoke at work. Should I cut these out when I stop smoking?' No. Don't worry about things you have already established as substitutions for smoking. Just focus on the possible danger of increasing the amount of substitution in the process of stopping smoking. If you usually eat popcorn at the cinema, for example, go ahead and do that, even if you only do it because the cinema is a no-smoking zone.

'When I smoke, I never eat breakfast (or lunch or dinner). Does this mean that I should never eat three meals a day after I have stopped smoking?' I recommend that for at least the first week of not smoking you deal with the desire to smoke you will feel at those times, and don't substitute (i.e. add) anything at all. After that, by all means eat something at these times, but remember, if you eat more food each day than you used to, for whatever reason, you are likely to gain weight. If you only used to eat one meal a day, then you could spread the equivalent amount over the whole day, eating smaller amounts at more frequent intervals. If you make this change after at least a week in your regular routine, it's less likely to be a choice that feeds your addiction.

'Will it help me to substitute nicotine gum?' I use the term substitution to mean something you do or consume instead of nicotine. In that sense, nicotine gum, lozenges or patches are not really a substitution: they are simply other ways of taking the same drug.

Nicotine replacement products could give you some confidence to start with, but using them can mean that the whole process just gets more drawn out.

A number of research studies have shown that nicotine replacement is hardly effective at all when used alone, and has only produced modest success in the long term when used together with regular group meetings.[3]

If you are very keen to use some form of nicotine replacement together with this book, I recommend you use the patches, because they bring nicotine into your body in a passive way. In other words, you don't consume anything in response to your desire to smoke.

'Does this mean I can't smoke, and now I can't eat either?' Deprivation is the underlying cause of substitution. If you believe you can't smoke you are more likely to want to eat to compensate and to reward yourself for the self-sacrifice you believe you are making. If you also believe you can't substitute either, you will feel very sorry for yourself until you start to rebel by eating or smoking – or both!

The helpful thing to remember about substitution is that you are not cutting out food and drink that you enjoy when you stop smoking: you are simply making sure you don't *increase* your eating and drinking, so you can identify and manage your desire to smoke. And don't forget – you don't *have to* do any of this at all.

The Value of Welcoming

It's likely you have satisfied your addictive hunger with cigarettes on many occasions in the past. You got into the habit of smoking instead of eating and then, when you stop smoking, it's easy to switch to eating instead of smoking. The desire to smoke and the desire to eat can become entwined, interchangeable and even indistinguishable from each other.

What this means is that, in order to stop smoking without gaining weight, it will be essential for you to make some choices to accept feeling your addictive desire to eat.

At first, the more aware you are of your desire to eat, the more you can be in control, but you won't need to watch out for substitutions for the rest of your life. Weight gain is always a possibility, of course, even for smokers, but it's when you first stop smoking and the addictive desire is at its strongest that it's most likely to be satisfied with substitutions.

The desire to smoke and the desire to eat can become entwined, interchangeable and even indistinguishable from each other.

I didn't gain weight when I stopped smoking, and although my weight has fluctuated over the years, it's fluctuated no more than when I smoked. In my own experience – both as an ex-smoker and as someone who has a tendency to overeat – smoking makes addictive eating more of a problem over the long term. It may seem a good idea to smoke a low-calorie cigarette instead of eating a snack, but in some sense it's the same addictive desire that is being reinforced when you do that.

When you stop trying to run away from your addictive desire and make that simple decision to face it and deal with it, you will find that many things start to work better for you.

This is the real value of welcoming, not only because you really do take and stay in control of your smoking, but also because, when you unconditionally accept the feeling of desire, you don't need to cover it up with any other compulsive behaviour.

If you follow this technique when you stop smoking, your weight gain, if any, will be slight. Just remember

Nathaniel Branden's words, that 'What is required for many of us is the courage to tolerate success without self-sabotage, until such time as we lose our fear of it and realise that it will not destroy us – and need not disappear'.

IN OTHER WORDS: CATHY

My weight is now around nine and a half stone and I have not put on any weight since I packed up smoking. I do remember wanting to eat more in the early days, and using the question: 'Would I be eating this if I was still smoking?' I believe that without that I would have eaten a lot more. One day in particular I felt haunted by a bar of chocolate I had in the fridge and I used The Outline a lot that day. I remember that it was tough, but I stayed with it and conquered it. Looking back on it now, I can see that day was a major turning point for me. I did have more desires to smoke after that but I knew it was up to me, it was my choice. I love knowing that, and until now, more than three years later, I haven't smoked. Full Stop is one of the best things I have ever done for myself.

CHAPTER 14

Staying Stopped for Good

When people will not weed their own minds, they are apt to be overrun with nettles.

HORACE WALPOLE

When you stop smoking you can expect to go through a couple of days of withdrawal, and after that, assuming you are managing it correctly, your desire to smoke will begin to diminish. It diminishes in *frequency* first of all, so you get longer gaps of time in between feeling the desire. Then, after a week or so, it begins to diminish in *intensity* as well, so that the sensations you feel will lessen and become more like strong thoughts.

Your expectation of how rapidly your desire should diminish is crucial to your acceptance of it, so it's helpful to keep things in perspective. Expect that your desire might be fairly frequent for about as many days as the number of years you spent smoking. If you look at it that way, the presence of the uncomfortable, unsatisfied desire will seem more reasonable.

Be careful if you make a comparison between smoking and other addictions you may have conquered. What makes smoking different, and in this regard more difficult, is that it gets so thoroughly integrated into your life, reinforced daily over a great many years. That tends to make the desire to smoke more persistent than almost any other addictive desire.

When you first stop smoking, think of the desire to smoke that you experience as being the result of the sum total of all the cigarettes you ever smoked.

The more you have smoked, the more persistent your desire to smoke will be. That's why, if you go on smoking, it will never get any easier for you to stop, and why it's best to get out of it as soon as you have the chance to do so.

Fading Desire and the 'Firsts'

For the first couple of days, while the desire is fairly constant, you will need to find an acceptable compromise between dealing with your desire to smoke and sometimes having your mind on something else. As the desire begins to lessen, you still need to use The Outline, see page 114, as soon as possible whenever you notice that your desire has reappeared.

After a few weeks, you may only feel the desire to smoke a few times in a day and it may only last a few moments, but it's still important to deal with it when it appears; otherwise you can fall back into your old addictive thinking.

One question that is often asked at this stage is: 'How do I know if the desire is really diminishing, or if I'm repressing it?' The answer depends on your attitude towards it.

You can be confident that you're not repressing your desire if you really are welcoming your experience of it. This means opening yourself up to it and letting yourself feel it. It may not be very strong and it may not last for very long, but if you are sincerely willing to feel it, it's not being repressed.

During the first few weeks of not smoking, you can expect to deal with some particularly strong feelings of desire because of a series of 'firsts'. A 'first' is the first time that you are in a particular situation where you used to smoke. There is an immediate connection that produces an intense desire. This is when you can see that the desire is coming from your memory of smoking.

When you have only just stopped smoking, the 'firsts' happen in rapid succession: the first time you finish a meal, the first time you get home from work, the first time you answer the phone, the first time you watch TV. Later, they happen less often, but can be surprisingly powerful: the first time you get angry or disappointed, the first time you go on holiday, the first time you visit a particular friend who smokes, or a certain place where you used to smoke.

As you continue to notice and manage the desire, you'll see it will fade in each situation. Even so, you may find that a more persistent desire is associated with certain sorts of situations. For some people, the strongest desire to smoke is always first thing in the morning; for others it's late at night. For some, the strongest desire to smoke happens when they are relaxing or out in the evening with friends; for others it's when they are working or when they are alone.

After a while, most of the associations will have faded simply because you have encountered them without smoking. Then, your desire to smoke will rarely, if ever, appear in that particular situation. You may even find yourself reflecting on a recent event and be surprised by the fact that you didn't think of smoking at the time.

After over 20 years of not smoking, I cannot say that I ever feel any desire to smoke at all. The situation in which I most often had a desire to smoke was when I was with good friends who smoked, at a dinner party for example. At those times it would seem to me that smoking a cigarette would be extremely enjoyable. My desire to smoke would last about 30 seconds, and I would welcome the mildly uncomfortable sensation, reminding myself that I prefer the better health and greater energy I have gained. Mostly, I really like being free from the compulsive, driven quality that characterises this addiction.

I know that I am not immune to the addiction, and I can return to smoking any time. And I am very sure that it's not worth risking even one puff! The bottom line for me is this: what if smoking one cigarette leads me back into smoking every day for the rest of my life? If there is even a slight chance of that, it's not worth the risk. And there is more than a slight chance, in my opinion.

Smokers Smoking

When you see other people smoking, expect to have a desire to smoke yourself. Being in the company of smokers produces some of the most persistent associations. Be very careful of this desire, because when you notice someone else smoking, you are likely to recall some of your favourite delusions, such as: 'they only smoke a few cigarettes', 'they do it because it's enjoyable', and 'it's innocent fun'.

If you feel envious of smokers, remind yourself that you have the option of going back to smoking yourself, but remember also the truth behind the delusion. First, although smokers only smoke one cigarette at a time, that cigarette is one of more than a hundred they go through every week. *Your desire to smoke looks like a desire for one cigarette, but know that, once satisfied, it is a desire for thousands.*

Smokers may look as though they are enjoying their cigarettes, although the chances are they are not. Either way, they are compelled to keep smoking them, because otherwise they would have an unsatisfied desire to smoke, and they don't know how to live with it without smoking.

Not only that, but smokers are in fact perpetually at the beginning of withdrawal, every time a cigarette is extinguished. And what is often not apparent is the guilt and fear they live with, their deteriorating state of health, their constant broken promises to stop, and their loss of self-esteem.

It's essential that you see your desire to smoke for what it is: the automatic, habitual memory of your addiction. Do not confuse it with wanting to return to a life of smoking.

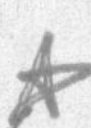

Over to You

If by now you have read the whole of this book, but you have not yet stopped smoking, you may be thinking, 'Is this it?'

A number of clients have told me that while attending my course, they found themselves with a sense of wanting something more. They also told me that they realised at the time that what they were wanting was to have stopping smoking done for them. What they really wanted was to be told to stop or somehow made to stop smoking. When they realised that, they also realised that the first decision to begin the process of stopping smoking was, ultimately, up to them. And when that thought clicked into place, they did choose to stop smoking, and began the process of learning how to stay stopped for good.

Stopping smoking is not a single event: it is a process of retraining your addicted mind.

If you have now stopped smoking, I suggest you keep reviewing this book, say once a week to begin with, and at least once a month for the first year of your life as an ex-smoker.

Stopping smoking is not a single event: it is a process of retraining your addicted mind. This takes time and it takes effort, but it is entirely possible for you to succeed completely. The longer you stay stopped, and the more deeply you involve yourself with the techniques in this book, the more likely you are to succeed.

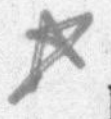

You cannot undo the past. But you can take control of the present. And so determine your future.

IN OTHER WORDS: JIMMY

I smoked upwards of 40 a day for 25 years, from the age of 15 to 40. Several people said: 'Jimmy will never stop smoking,' in those words, while I was a smoker.

I did not want to stop, but thought I had to. I convinced myself that I was a 'natural smoker', but increasingly feared illness.

I had tried acupuncture, hypnosis and willpower alone, with temporary success. I chewed nicotine chewing gum for a year. I stopped, had a jaw like a wrestler, but started smoking again days after stopping chewing.

Full Stop worked, and more than three years later I am still an ex-smoker. I still feel liberated and it's wonderful.

Of course, I still feel the desire to smoke, and I still welcome it. Since doing the course, my life has had its share of problems. One thought that I find vital at moments of crisis is that if I smoke, I'll just have another problem on my hands.

Your Plan for Stopping

Step by Step

1 Read this book, all the way through, at least once. Keep your copy so you can refer to it for some time to come.

2 Writing notes and personal insights in a journal can be helpful for some people. At least write down the reasons why you want to stop smoking, and, after you've stopped, add notes on anything you like about not smoking. A written record can help you because it's very easy to forget what's at stake. Most people take things for granted after not smoking for a while, and can even begin to romanticise smoking as 'the good old days'. Often it's only when they've returned to smoking that they remember exactly what a misery it was for them.

3 Pick a date to quit. If you choose a date that has a special significance for you, you might be more likely to remember it and keep to it. However, don't completely rule out the possibility of quitting spontaneously when an opportunity has arisen: visiting the doctor, for example, or starting a new job.

4 Practise for up to five days before your quit date. This is not an essential part of quitting but can be a useful stepping-stone, provided it's just for a few days. This is how to practise:

- Deal with each desire to smoke in the present time by telling yourself: 'I have a desire to smoke and I have the freedom to smoke.' Then make a choice either to smoke or to accept that desire to smoke for that moment.
- If you choose to smoke, wait for the next desire and make another choice.
- Keep your cigarettes with you.
- If you are not feeling your desire to smoke at least as often as you normally would, induce the desire. The more choices you make not to smoke while you are feeling the desire, the better.
- Don't establish a pattern of substitution. You are much better off smoking at this stage than creating an additional problem by eating or drinking more. See Chapter 13 for more on this.
- Keep it all to yourself.
- Don't get discouraged by the smoking you do at this practice stage. You are just testing the waters.
- During this practice you may get the impression that all you are doing is delaying smoking. This is fine; your purpose here is to practise managing your desire to smoke.

5 Quitting.

- When you get to your quit date, you stop smoking entirely by using The Outline (see page 192). Essentially, what you will be adding is: 'One puff and I'll be smoking,' which takes you from practising to stopping.
- Chapters 6 and 9 would be good to review at this point.
- It can be very helpful to keep quiet about having stopped for as long as possible. If anyone notices and asks, say something vague about cutting down and change the subject if you can.

6 Staying stopped.

- Make a point of reviewing this book from time to time. You could simply pick it up now and then and read a page or two at a time. Many people have told me they keep their copy in the loo!
- Your desire to smoke will begin to fade during your first week of not smoking, but can return at full strength, often without warning. Stay in practice with managing your desire from time to time (see below), especially during the first year after stopping.
- Expect to come up with every excuse under the sun to smoke a cigarette. Look out for: 'that wasn't so bad, I could quit again any time' and 'I've done so well I'm sure I could handle one now'.
- Take the idea of smoking again very seriously, being careful not to develop a cycle of frequent stopping and starting. Apart from the fact that it tends to take over your life, you end up devaluing quitting so much that it becomes meaningless. Then you give up giving up and resign yourself to a life of smoking.

Troubleshooting

Managing Your Desire to Smoke

Your long-term success depends on one skill: your ability to manage your desire to smoke while you are feeling it. Here's a summary:

- *Pay attention* to your thoughts and feelings of desire. Notice any physical sensations of desire, giving them your full attention and relaxing with them as much as possible.

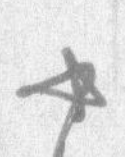

- *Let go* of anxiety about failure by staying in the present time. You don't need to know if you'll smoke later on; maybe you will and maybe you won't. You can only take control in the present time.
- *Connect* with choice: 'I'm free to smoke.' Know that you have access to cigarettes so that this choice is real.
- *Consider* the consequences of the choices open to you.
- *Choose* either to satisfy the desire (= return to smoking) or to accept it (= feel it).
- *Your choice to accept* the desire is your choice to feel uncomfortable and unsatisfied. Know that this is your healing process. By accepting this feeling, you succeed at quitting, gain an improved quality of life and allow your desire to smoke to fade away.
- *Resolve* any conflict by asking yourself: am I willing to accept this uncomfortable feeling of desire or would I rather spend the rest of my life smoking?

The Outline

How to Make a Choice

I have a desire to smoke

I have the freedom to smoke

One puff and I'll be smoking

Either:

I choose to return to smoking

Or:

For now, I choose to accept this desire

So I can enjoy these benefits from not smoking . . .

Feeling Deprived

This is the number-one obstacle to long-term success, so consider the following:

- *Notice* any symptoms of deprivation and *do not tolerate them for any length of time.* They are dangerous as they are likely to lead you back to smoking.
- *Symptoms* of deprivation are any negative emotions over and above those you would usually feel when you were smoking. For many people these are *extra*: irritability, anger, sadness, anxiety, panic, apathy, lethargy, self-pity, loss and/or grief. They are often accompanied by more persistent, prolonged and intense cravings.
- *Identify the cause.* These negative reactions come from feeling *as if* you were locked into one irrevocable decision never to smoke again.
- *Release* these feelings immediately by connecting with your freedom of choice: 'I don't have to do this – I'm free to return to smoking any time.' See Chapter 4 for more on this. If a sense of deprivation is very tough for you to overcome, completing the written exercise on page 131 will be a very good idea. Repeat this exercise at least a few times a week.
- *Spend time* considering the fact that you have got choices and what making various choices would mean to you.
- *Stay in the now.* Feelings of deprivation are often created by a strong fear of failure. The remedy is to train yourself to only make your choices in the present time as far as not smoking is concerned. See Chapter 5 for more on this and remember it's always a case of 'so far, so good'. Just give it a try. See how long you can keep it up and you might be very surprised!

The Full Stop Technique: An Overview

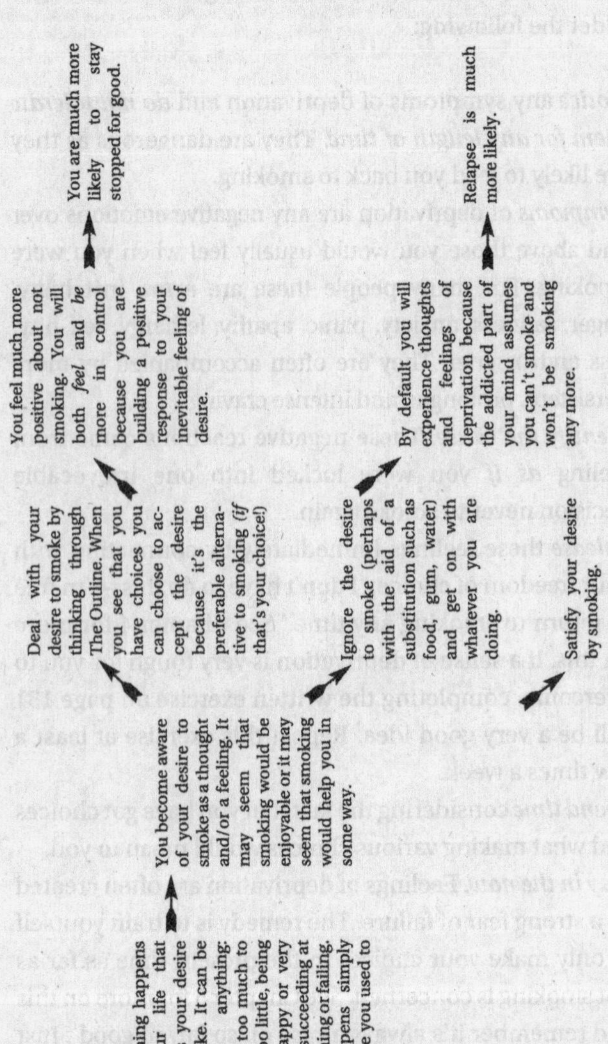

Something happens in your life that triggers your desire to smoke. It can be almost anything: having too much to do or too little, being very happy or very upset, succeeding at something or failing. It happens simply because you used to smoke.
You become aware of your desire to smoke as a thought and/or a feeling. It may seem that smoking would be enjoyable or it may seem that smoking would help you in some way.
Deal with your desire to smoke by thinking through The Outline. When you see that you have choices you can choose to accept the desire because it's the preferable alternative to smoking (if that's your choice!)
You feel much more positive about not smoking. You will both feel and be more in control because you are building a positive response to your inevitable feeling of desire.
You are much more likely to stay stopped for good.
Ignore the desire to smoke (perhaps with the aid of a substitution such as food, gum, water) and get on with whatever you are doing.
By default you will experience thoughts and feelings of deprivation because the addicted part of your mind assumes you can't smoke and won't be smoking any more.
Relapse is much more likely.
Satisfy your desire by smoking.
For the vast majority of ex-smokers, these first two stages are inevitable, unavoidable and automatic.
The rest is not inevitable because you have a choice: either ignore the desire or deal with it effectively using The Outline.

Further Help

For information on telephone counselling, you can reach Gillian Riley through her website www.eatingless.com. Gillian currently leads seminars on taking control of overeating. Her other books are:

Eating Less: Say Goodbye to Overeating (Vermilion, 1999, 2005)
Quitting Smoking (Gill & Macmillan/Newleaf, 2001)
Willpower! (Vermilion, 2003)

References

Chapter 2

1 Jarvis, M., *Nicotine Replacement: A Critical Evaluation* (1988), p.146. In another experiment, volunteer smokers were given pills to take regularly during a normal smoking day and, at the same time, were asked to keep a record of when they smoked. 'They were unaware of the content of the pills, which were identified only by the day and time they were to be taken. On some days the smokers took nothing but sugar pills, but on other days they took doses of nicotine equivalent to that ingested by smoking. On average, they smoked twenty-four cigarettes on the days they were taking the sugar pills and twenty-two cigarettes on the nicotine days.' Jarvik, Glick and Nakamura, 'Inhibition of cigarette smoking by orally administered nicotine', *Clinical Pharmacology and Therapeutics* (1970), 11: 574–76.

2 Injections of nicotine were given to 35 volunteers. 'Smokers almost invariably thought the sensation pleasant, and given an adequate dose, were disinclined to smoke for a time thereafter. After a course of eighty injections of nicotine, an injection was preferred to a cigarette.' Johnston, L., 'Tobacco Smoking and Nicotine', *The Lancet* (1942), p.742.

3 From the last cigarette smoked, the amount of nicotine in the blood stream drops by half every two hours. After 12 hours, very little nicotine is left. Benowitz, N., Jacob, P., Jones, R., and Rosenberg, J., 'Interindividual variability in the metabolism and cardiovascular effects of nicotine in man', *Journal of Pharmacology and Experimental Therapeutics* (1982), 221:368–372.

Chapter 3

1 'Behaviour modification techniques (relaxation, rewards and punishment, avoiding "trigger" situations, etc.), in group or individual sessions led by a psychologist, have an effect that is statistically significant but not greater than simple advice by a physician (2%).' Law, M., Tang, J., 'An analysis of the effectiveness of interventions intended to help people stop smoking', *Archives of Internal Medicine* (1995), 155 (18):1933–41.

'Despite increasing popular interest in acupuncture as a treatment technique, it has not been demonstrated that acupuncture is able to promote smoking cessation . . . Past reviews of smoking modification research indicate that aversive techniques largely have failed to help people to quit smoking . . . From my review of over 50 reports, comments and critiques of the use of hypnosis to control smoking, I conclude that hypnosis produces only modest results.' *Review and Evaluation of Smoking Cessation Methods: US and Canada (1978–1985)*, US Department of Health and Human Services, National Institutes of Health, Washington, DC.

'Acupuncture and nicotine gum were effective in helping smokers to stop smoking during the first month but did not reduce the tendency to relapse after that time.' 'Helping people to stop smoking: randomised comparison of groups being treated with acupuncture and nicotine gum compared with control group', *British Medical Journal* (1985), 291:1538–1539.

Chapter 6

1 Research on this, published in the journal *Addictive Behaviors* (15:105–114, 1990), followed 129 smokers after they had stopped. Of those who smoked even one puff, 88 per cent returned to full-time smoking. On average they smoked their second cigarette nine days later, and took six weeks to return to daily smoking.

2 According to research published in the *British Medical Journal*, 53 per cent of smokers say they expect to quit within the next two years, when in fact, just 6 per cent manage to do that.

Chapter 7

1 Skrabanek, Petr, and McCormick, James, *Follies and Fallacies in Medicine* (1989), Tarragon Press.

Chapter 8

1 Reported in *The Guardian*, September 2004.

2 According to research published in the *International Journal of Dermatology* (November 2002), it is thought that toxins in cigarettes impair the elasticity of skin, so that lines on the faces of smokers are twice as deep as those on non-smokers of the same age.

3 Johnston, L., 'Tobacco Smoking and Nicotine', *The Lancet* (1942), p.742.

4 Siana, J. E., Rex, S., and Gottrup, F., 'The effect of cigarette smoking on wound healing', *Scand. J. Plas. Reconstr. Surgery* (1990), 23:207–209.

Chapter 9

1 *The Health Consequences of Smoking: Nicotine Addiction* (1988), US Department of Health and Human Services.

Chapter 10

1 'Withdrawal symptoms were less reliably alleviated [by nicotine gum]. These included depression, anxiety/tension, difficulty concentrating, restlessness and the urge to smoke.' *Nicotine Addiction: The Health Consequences of Smoking* (1988), US Department of Health and Human Services. Report of the Surgeon General, p.208. 'Five symptoms – dizziness, alertness, frustration, feeling miserable, and disorientation – were not affected by nicotine relative to placebo.' Pomerleau, O. F., and

Pomerleau, C. S., *Nicotine Replacement: A Critical Evaluation* (1988), Alan R. Liss, NY, p.116. Another study demonstrates the same point in a different way: 'The de-nicotinised cigarettes were equivalent [to regular cigarettes] in reducing acute withdrawal symptoms.' Butschky, M., Bailey, D., Henningfield, J., Pickworth, W., 'Smoking without nicotine delivery decreases withdrawal in 12-hour abstinent smokers', *Pharmacology, Biochemistry and Behaviour* (1995), 50(1):91–6.

Chapter 12

1 '. . . over fifty million working days were lost each year due to smoking-related illness and the likely cost in terms of lost production was estimated to be between £2,200 million and £3,200 million'. HoC *Hansard*, Col.349W 11/3/91.

Chapter 13

1 'Time course of cigarette withdrawal symptoms during four weeks of treatment with nicotine chewing gum' (1987), *Addictive Behaviors* 12:199–203.

2 This study was published in the *International Journal of Obesity* in 2005, 29: 236–243.

3 'One of the more reliable findings about nicotine gum has been that it is only marginally efficacious, if at all, when prescribed in the absence of a context for behaviour change.' Pomerleau, O.F., Pomerleau, C.S., *Nicotine Replacement: A Critical Evaluation* (1988), Alan R. Liss, NY, p.285; Campbell, I., Lyons, E., and Prescott, R., 'Stopping Smoking: Do nicotine chewing-gum and postal encouragement add to doctors' advice?', *The Practitioner* (1987), 231:114–117; Jamrozik, K., Fowler, G., Vessey, M., Wald, N., 'Placebo controlled trial of nicotine chewing gum in general practice', *British Medical Journal* (1984), 289:794–797.

Acknowledgements

I would like to thank Joe Zeitchick, who taught me how to stop smoking, and Drs K. Bradford Brown and W. Roy Whitten, who helped me broaden my understanding of the processes involved.

Peter Holmes, Peggy Holmes and Patricia Allison have worked with similar techniques and I am grateful to them for their input over the years.

Many thanks go to everyone who helped in various ways with the writing of this book, especially Gillian Barnett and David Templer. Thanks also to my clients who contributed their own stories about stopping smoking.

About the Author

A former smoker and overeater, **Gillian Riley** has been teaching her successful techniques for stopping smoking and eating less since 1982.

Gillian led her first seminars on stopping smoking in the United States, where she lived for 17 years. In 1984 she returned to her home town of London and has been living and working in the UK since then. Gillian led seminars on how to stop smoking for about 14 years, supporting her clients with telephone counselling for many months after thay had quit. This is where she really understood what it takes to stay stopped

During follow-up counselling with ex-smokers, she soon realised that for many of them the biggest challenge they faced was staying in control of their eating. After working one-to-one with these clients for some time, Gillian developed techniques and a seminar to offer to anyone who experiences loss of control over food.

How To Stop Smoking And Stay Stopped For Good is widely used in smoking clinics within the National Health Service in the UK. Gillian no longer runs seminars for smokers. Since 1996 she has delivered a number of training seminars for professionals in the National Health Service on how to help smokers quit. Gillian introduced the Eating Less seminars in 1997, publishing an accompanying book.

Gillian has been a guest on television and radio, including BBC1, GMTV, ITV, Talk Radio and the BBC World Service. Gillian is also a regular guest speaker at *Ragdale Hall Health Hydro* in Leicestershire, where she gives introductory talks on taking control of overeating.

Index

Also by Gillian Riley

Eating Less
Say goodbye to overeating

Are you caught up in a cycle of binge eating and dieting?
Do you think about food most of the day?
Do you feel guilty about what you eat?
If so, *Eating Less* is the book for you.

As anyone who has ever been on a diet knows, they simply don't work: once you stop, the weight piles back on. *Eating Less* is not about dieting; instead it places emphasis where it belongs – on healthy eating and eating less.

This revised and updated edition offers you a unique and inspiring solution that:

- Introduces you to practical techniques that you can apply in your daily life
- Shows you how to set your own limits on food without feeling deprived or becoming rebellious
- Gives you the ability to develop greater control by helping you to overcome addictive behaviour

So, simply start *Eating Less* and see your weight fall off – and stay off.

Also by Gillian Riley

Willpower!

Break bad habits, stick to your true goals and create the life you want

You already have willpower. Everyone does. All you need is to learn how to use it.

With just a little practice, willpower can work even when you don't feel inspired, even when you are faced with your strongest temptations. And the wonderful news is that willpower isn't something that gets handed out to some and not others. It's simply a matter of understanding how to access it and unlock its potential. When you do you'll see just how liberating, exciting and rewarding using willpower can be. Very soon, rather than being your own worst enemy, you'll become your own best friend.

Use the brilliant strategies in this book to:

- Overcome addictive behaviours
- Quit smoking
- Take control of overeating
- Achieve your dreams
- Enhance your life

With a little belief, some confidence and the techniques laid out in this revolutionary book, you'll soon discover just how strong your willpower can be.

☐	Eating Less	9780091902476	£7.99
☐	Willpower!	9780091887698	£8.99

FREE POSTAGE AND PACKING

Overseas customers allow £2.00 per paperback.

BY PHONE: 01624 677237

BY POST: Random House Books
c/o Bookpost, PO Box 29, Douglas
Isle of Man, IM99 1BQ

BY FAX: 01624 670923

BY EMAIL: bookshop@enterprise.net

Cheques (payable to Bookpost)
and credit cards accepted.

Prices and availability subject to change without notice.
Allow 28 days for delivery.
When placing your order, please mention if you do not
wish to receive any additional information.

www.randomhouse.co.uk

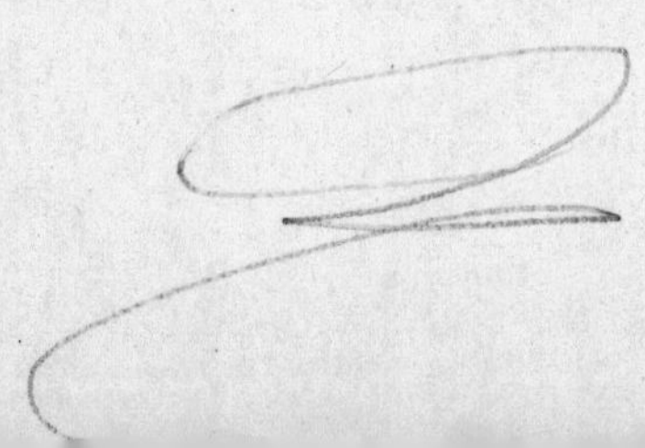

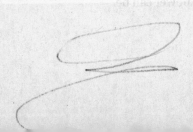